Erectile Dysfunction

A Clinical Guide

by

Roger Kirby MA MD FRCS (Urol) FEBU
*Consultant Urologist, Department of Urology,
St. George's Hospital, London, UK*

Culley Carson III MD
*Professor and Chief, Division of Urology, Department of Surgery,
University of North Carolina School of Medicine, Chapel Hill, USA*

and

Irwin Goldstein MD
*Professor of Urology, Boston University School of Medicine,
Boston, USA*

with contributions from

Ahmed Fawzy MD FACS
*Co-director of Research, Urologic Institute of New Orleans,
Gretna, USA*

Kevin McVary MD
*Associate Professor, Department of Urology,
Northwestern University Medical School, Chicago, USA*

I S I S
MEDICAL
M E D I A

© 1999 by Isis Medical Media Ltd.
59 St Aldates
Oxford OX1 1ST, UK

First published 1999

British Library Cataloguing in Publication Data.
A catalogue record for this title is available from
the British Library.

ISBN 1 901865 24 X

Kirby, R. (Roger)
Erectile Dysfunction: A Clinical Guide
Roger Kirby, Culley Carson, Irwin Goldstein (authors)

Always refer to the manufacturer's Prescribing
Information before prescribing drugs cited in this book.

Medical writing by
Christine McKillop PhD

Artwork by
Dee McLean

Typeset by
Creative Associates, Oxford

Produced by Phoenix Offset, HK
Printed in China

Distributed in the USA by
Books International, Inc., P.O. Box 605,
Herndon, VA 20172, USA

Distributed in the rest of the world by
Plymbridge Distributors Ltd., Estover Road,
Plymouth, PL6 7PY, UK

Contents

Chapter 1
Epidemiology

Erectile dysfunction (ED), or impotence as it was previously known, is defined as the consistent inability to achieve and/or maintain an erection sufficient for satisfactory sexual activity. The causes of ED are frequently multifactorial, with psychological, neurological, endocrinological, vascular, traumatic and iatrogenic components described. ED is usually divided into organic and psychogenic, according to the main contributors to the dysfunction. Very little high-quality epidemiological investigation of this disorder has been undertaken, so the relative importance of the various causes of ED is unknown at present. Potential risk factors have been identified, however, and include ageing, smoking, hypertension, hyperlipidaemia, diabetes mellitus, depression and vascular disease, as well as a variety of drugs.

■ ED, or impotence as it was previously known, is defined as the consistent inability to achieve and/or maintain an erection sufficient for satisfactory sexual activity.

■ Quality of life

Although ED is considered a benign disorder, it may have a dramatic impact on the quality of life of many men as well as their sexual partners. It is difficult to assess the precise effect of ED on quality of life because the dysfunction may be partly a result of a pre-existing psychological problem, which complicates interpretation. Nevertheless, ED often results in anxiety, depression and lack of self-esteem and self-confidence, which in themselves can perpetuate the disorder.

Emotional disturbances are often overlooked in quantitative research as most sex-related questionnaires

■ ED often results in anxiety, depression and lack of self-esteem and self-confidence.

focus on functional ability. This is changing, however, with the recent development of instruments that measure the quality of life specific to ED.

■ Prevalence

The prevalence of ED has been studied through the use of questionnaires. One such questionnaire which has been developed recently is the Brief Sexual Function Inventory (SFI) (Table 1.1). This includes questions on sexual drive, erection, ejaculation, perceptions of problems in each of these areas and overall satisfaction. Another similar questionnaire, the International Index of Erectile Dysfunction, includes questions on erectile function, orgasmic function, sexual desire, intercourse satisfaction and overall satisfaction (see Chapter 3).

A particular problem with assessing the prevalence of ED relates to the probability of a man truthfully declaring the extent and impact of his ED. Although some couples may accept reduced function as a natural part of ageing, others will be concerned and upset. Such facets of sexuality will have a strong influence on which men will admit to the interviewer that they have ED.

■ The Massachusetts Male Ageing Study found that among 1209 men the mean probability of some degree of ED was 52%.

The most useful and comprehensive study of the epidemiology of ED at present is the Massachusetts Male Ageing Study (MMAS), conducted between 1987 and 1989. This cross-sectional, random sample survey of health status and related issues was conducted in men between the ages of 40 and 70 years in the Boston area of Massachusetts. Analysis of data on 1209 men indicated that the mean probability of some degree of ED was 52.0 ± 1.3%. This could be divided according to the degree of ED into:

Table 1.1. The Brief Sexual Function Inventory	0	1	2	3	4
Sexual drive 1. During the past 30 days, on how many days have you felt sexual desire?	No days	Only a few days	Some days	Most days	Almost every day
2. During the past 30 days, how would you rate your level of sexual desire?	None at all	Low	Medium	Medium high	High
Erections 3. Over the past 30 days, how often have you had partial full erections when you were sexually stimulated in any way?	Not at all	A few times	Fairly often	Usually	Always
4. Over the past 30 days, how often were your erections firm enough to have sexual intercourse?	Not at all	A few times	Fairly often	Usually	Always
5. How much difficulty did you have in getting an erection during the last 30 days?	Did not get erections at all	A lot of difficulty	Some difficulty	Little difficulty	No difficulty
Ejaculation 6. Over the past 30 days, how much difficulty have you had in ejaculating when you have been sexually stimulated?	Have had no sexual stimulation in the past month	A lot of difficulty	Some difficulty	Little difficulty	No difficulty
7. Over the past 30 days, how much concern did you have over the amount of semen you ejaculated?	Did not climax	Big problem	Medium problem	Small problem	No problem
Problem assessment 8. In the past 30 days, to what extent have you considered a lack of sex drive to be a problem?	Big problem	Medium problem	Small problem	Very small problem	No problem
9. In the past 30 days, to what extent have you considered your ability to get and keep an erection a problem?	Big problem	Medium problem	Small problem	Very small problem	No problem
10. In the past 30 days, to what extent have you considered your ejaculation to be a problem?	Big problem	Medium problem	Small problem	Very small problem	No problem
Overall satisfaction 11. Overall, during the past 30 days, how satisfied have you been with your sex life?	Very dissatisfied	Mostly dissatisfied	Neutral or mixed	Mostly satisfied	Very satisfied

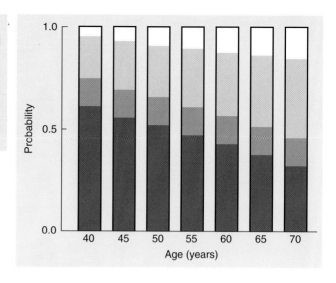

Figure 1.1.
Relationship between age and degree of ED in the MMAS.
■ None; ■ minimal; ▨ moderate; ☐ complete.
Reproduced with permission from Feldman H *et al*. J Urol 1994;151:54–61.

- Minimal, 17.2%
- Moderate, 25.2%
- Complete, 9.6%.

■ The probability of ED was found to increase with age, from 5.1% at age 50 to 15% at age 70.

Between the fifth and seventh decades, the probability of complete ED almost tripled from 5.1% to 15% (Fig. 1.1). In all, 60% of men were potent in their fifth decade compared with only 33% at 70 years.

■ Risk factors

Vascular disease

Vascular disease of various types has been associated with ED, including:

- Myocardial infarction (MI)

■ Alterations in vascular haemodynamics are believed to be the most common cause of organic ED.

- Coronary artery disease
- Cerebrovascular accidents
- Peripheral vascular disease
- Hypertension
- Atherosclerosis/dyslipidaemia.

Indeed, alterations in the vascular haemodynamics are believed to be the most common cause of organic ED. In men with MI aged 31–86 years, 64% were shown to have ED, while in another study, 57% of men undergoing coronary bypass surgery were found to have the condition. The incidence of ED in men with severe peripheral vascular disease has been estimated at 80%.

Cigarette smoking

Cigarette smoking has been identified as a risk factor for (vascular) ED. In the MMAS among subjects with treated heart disease, the age-adjusted probabilities of complete ED were:

- Smokers, 56%
- Non-smokers, 21%.

Similar results were observed in treated hypertensives:

- Smokers, 20%
- Non-smokers, 8.5%.

The study also found that the effects of drugs were exacerbated by smoking, with the age-adjusted probability of complete impotence being increased in those taking the following medications:

- Cardiac medication: from 14% to 41%
- Antihypertensive medications: from 7.5% to 21%
- Vasodilators: from 21% to 52%.

In general, however, an overall effect of current smoking on ED was not noted, with an 11% incidence of complete ED in smokers compared with 9.3% of non-smokers. Among current smokers, the probability of ED showed no dose-dependency with current smoking or lifetime cigarette consumption.

Diabetes

In the MMAS, the age-adjusted probability of complete ED was three times higher in men with diabetes.

> ■ Cigarette smoking is a risk factor for ED in patients with treated heart disease and hypertension; however, overall, cigarette smoking does not increase the incidence of ED.

■ The prevalence of ED in diabetics is 35–75% and increases with age.

Studies on diabetics have consistently shown a higher prevalence of ED, with estimates ranging from 35% to 75%. It has also been reported that ED in diabetics is age-related, with a 15% incidence at age 30–34, increasing to 55% at age 60. Of those diabetic men who will develop ED, 50% do so within 5–10 years of the diagnosis of diabetes. Those men with peripheral neuropathy, retinopathy, hypertension and renal failure are more likely to have ED.

High density lipoprotein-cholesterol

■ The probability of ED has been shown to be inversely related to the level of HDL-C.

In the MMAS, the probability of ED was inversely related to the level of high density lipoprotein-cholesterol (HDL-C). For younger men (40–55 years) the age-adjusted probability of moderate ED increased from 6.7% to 25% as HDL-C decreased from 90 to 30 mg/dl. In older subjects (56–70 years), the probability of complete ED increased from near zero to 16% as HDL-C decreased from 90 to 30 mg/dl. No association was found between total cholesterol and incidence of ED. Laboratory studies, however, have shown decreased corpus cavernosum smooth muscle function with elevated cholesterol level.

Surgery or trauma

■ Surgery or trauma affecting either the nervous system or interfering with the blood supply to the penis are associated with increased incidence of ED.

Surgery or trauma affecting either the nervous system or interfering with the blood supply to the penis are associated with increased incidence of ED (Table 1.2). Severe pelvis fractures, causing disruption of the prostato-membranous urethra, has been associated with a more than 50% incidence of ED. It has recently been suggested that erectile difficulties in young men can be the result of previous crossbar injuries incurred in bicycling accidents or repetitive injury from bicycle seats.

Table 1.2. Surgery and trauma associated with ED

Neurological	Head trauma/surgery Spinal cord trauma/surgery Retroperitoneal lymph node dissection
Vascular	Aortoiliac bypass Aortofemoral bypass
Gastroenterological	Abdominal-perineal resection Proctocolectomy Low anterior resection
Pelvis	Pelvic trauma Pelvic irradiation Pelvic lymphadenectomy
Urological	Implantation of I^{125} into the prostate Radical prostatectomy Cystoprostatectomy Perineal urethroplasty Open prostatectomy Bilateral orchiectomy Transurethral urethrotomy Transurethral sphincterotomy Transurethral prostatectomy

Drugs

Drug-related ED is common, although evidence for certain associations is based only on case reports and personal case series. Medication-induced ED has been estimated to occur in 25% of patients in a medical outpatient clinic. Of the medications listed in Table 1.3, thiazide diuretics are the most common cause of ED because of their common usage. Certain classes of antihypertensive agent are associated with ED in 4% to 40% of patients. They act directly at the corporal level (e.g. calcium channel blockers) or indirectly by reducing systemic blood pressure, which is important for the development of penile rigidity. Oestrogens, luteinizing hormone-releasing hormone (LHRH) agonists, H_2 antagonists and spironolactone cause

■ A number of drugs have been associated with causing ED.

7

Table 1.3. Drugs associated with ED

Diuretics	Thiazides Spironolactone
Antihypertensives	Methyldopa Clonidine Reserpine β-blockers Guanethidine Verapamil
Cardiac/Circulatory	Clofibrate Gemfibrozil Digoxin
Tranquilizers	Phenothiazines Butyrophenones
Antidepressants	Tricyclic antidepressants Monoamine oxidase inhibitors Lithium Selective serotonin re-uptake inhibitors, e.g. Prozac
H_2 antagonists	Cimetidine Ranitidine
Hormones	Oestrogens Progesterone Corticosteroids Cyproterone acetate 5α-reductase inhibitors Luteinizing hormone-releasing hormone agonists
Cytotoxic agents	Cyclophosphamide Methotrexate Roferon-A
Anticholinergics	Disopyramide Anticonvulsants
Recreational	Alcohol Cocaine Marijuana

ED due to their antiandrogen activity. The antidepressants alter central nervous system mechanisms. Digoxin induces ED via blockade of the

Na-K-ATPase pump, resulting in a net increase in intracellular Ca and a subsequent increase in tone of corporal smooth muscle. Drugs used for the treatment of prostate cancer such as LHRH analogues almost invariably result in ED by causing hypogonadism.

Chronic illness
Renal and hepatic failure
Chronic renal failure can cause ED in up to 40% of men affected. The mechanism by which this occurs is probably multifactorial, involving endocrinological, neuropathic and vascular factors. Men on chronic dialysis have elevated prolactin and diminished testosterone levels. These endocrine abnormalities may be reversed by renal transplantation, as well as treatment with bromocriptine. A high incidence of veno-occlusive dysfunction has also been identified in this group of men.

> ■ Chronic renal failure can cause ED in up to 40% of men, while hepatic failure due to alcohol-induced liver cirrhosis can result in ED in 50% of men.

In patients with hepatic failure, ED can affect as many as 50% of those with alcohol-induced liver cirrhosis. The extent of the dysfunction also depends on the cause and severity of the liver failure.

Pulmonary disease
A 30% incidence of ED has been observed in men with chronic obstructive pulmonary disease, but who had normal peripheral and penile pulses.

Neurological disorders
Stroke, spinal cord injury, peripheral neuropathy, brain and spinal tumours, Alzheimer's disease and multiple sclerosis (MS) can all give rise to ED. An 85% incidence of ED has been recorded in men following a stroke and a 71% incidence in men with MS.

> ■ A variety of neurological disorders can give rise to ED.

Summary

■ Erectile dysfunction (ED) is defined as the consistent inability to achieve and/or maintain an erection sufficient for satisfactory sexual intercourse.

■ Although ED is usually considered a benign disorder, it may have a dramatic impact on the quality of life of not only many men, but also their sexual partners.

■ Potential risk factors include: ageing, vascular disease, cigarette smoking, diabetes, hyperlipidaemia, surgery/trauma, depression and alcohol.

■ The Massachusetts Male Ageing Study found that among 1209 men the mean probability of some degree of ED was 52%.

■ The degree of ED could be classified as minimal (17.2%), moderate (25.2%), or complete (9.6%).

■ The probability of ED was found to increase with age, from 5.1% at age 50 to 15% at age 70.

Chapter 2
Anatomy, physiology and pathophysiology

■ Anatomy
Anatomy of the penis

The penis consists of three cylindrical erectile bodies: two paired corpora cavernosa and the corpus spongiosum; the urethra lies within the latter (Fig. 2.1). Forming the walls of the two corpora cavernosa and the corpus spongiosum are the tunica albuginea and the corpus spongiosum albuginea, respectively. A thick elastic layer, the Buck's fascia, surrounds these structures and is firmly attached to the tunica albuginea. The remaining layers of the penis consist of subcutaneous cellular tissue, the Colles' fascia or superficial penile fascia and the skin.

■ The penis consists of three cylindrical erectile bodies: two paired corpora cavernosa and the corpus spongiosum.

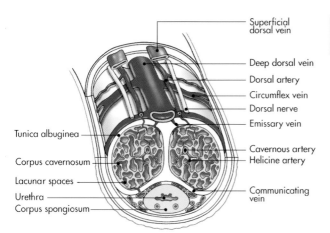

Figure 2.1.
A cross-section of the penis.

Superficial dorsal vein
Deep dorsal vein
Dorsal artery
Circumflex vein
Dorsal nerve
Emissary vein
Cavernous artery
Helicine artery
Communicating vein
Tunica albuginea
Corpus cavernosum
Lacunar spaces
Urethra
Corpus spongiosum

The corpora cavernosa make up the bulk of the penis and communicate for three-quarters of their length through a common medial septum that separates them. The septum is composed of multiple strands of elastic tissue and is perforated. Consequently, the two corpora can be considered a single blood space from a physiological viewpoint.

The corpus spongiosum contains the urethra and lies in the ventral groove formed by the two corpora cavernosa and traverses the length of the penis. At its proximal end it forms a bulb that is attached to the urogenital diaphragm. The urethra passes through this diaphragm and passes to the bladder. At the distal end, the corpus spongiosum expands to form the sensitive glans penis.

■ The erectile tissue is comprised of a lattice of vascular sinusoids surrounded by trabeculae of smooth muscle.

The erectile tissue is comprised of a lattice of vascular sinusoids surrounded by trabeculae of smooth muscle. The sinusoidal or lacunar spaces in the spongiosum are larger than those in the cavernosal bodies; there is also less smooth muscle present.

The skin over the penis is loosely adherent and highly flexible, allowing it to expand to permit an erection. At the distal end of the penis, the skin is attached to the corona of the glans and reflected forwards to form the prepuce or foreskin.

Vascular anatomy
Arterial supply

■ The main blood supply to the penis is derived from the pudendal artery, a branch of the internal iliac artery.

The blood supply to the penis derives mainly from the pudendal artery, which is a branch of the internal iliac artery. At the root of the penis, the pudendal artery becomes the common penile artery, which then gives off four branches (Fig. 2.2):

- Cavernosal artery
- Dorsal artery

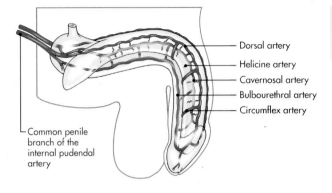

Figure 2.2.
The arterial supply to the penis.

Dorsal artery
Helicine artery
Cavernosal artery
Bulbourethral artery
Circumflex artery

Common penile branch of the internal pudendal artery

- Bulbar artery
- Urethral artery.

The cavernosal arteries run down the centre of each corpus cavernosum providing the main blood supply to the penis. They give off multiple corkscrew-shaped branches called helicine arteries that open directly into the lacunar spaces (Fig. 2.3). The helicine artery acts as a reactive blood vessel, which under the influence of the surrounding muscle, can induce a marked variability in resistance to vascular blood flow into the lacunar spaces.

The paired dorsal arteries travel along the dorsal surface of each corpora beneath the Buck's fascia to the

■ Cavernosal arteries run down the centre of each corpus cavernosum; they give off multiple helicine arteries, which open directly into the lacunar spaces.

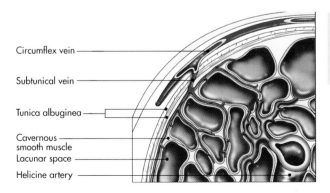

Circumflex vein
Subtunical vein
Tunica albuginea
Cavernous smooth muscle
Lacunar space
Helicine artery

Figure 2.3.
Arterial supply to the penis: opening of the helicine artery into the lacunar spaces.

13

glans penis. Up to 10 circumflex branches are given off and pass over the lateral surface of the corpora; these contribute to the blood supply to the corpora spongiosum and urethra. The terminal branches, in providing a blood supply, are responsible for the distension of the glans during erection.

The bulbar artery is a short artery that provides blood to the proximal end of the urethra and the Cowper's glands. The remainder of the urethra receives its blood supply from the urethral artery, as does the corpus spongiosum.

Venous drainage

■ The main venous drainage of the erectile tissue is via the deep dorsal, crural and cavernosal veins.

Venous drainage of the penis occurs through three systems (Fig. 2.4):

- Superficial
- Intermediate
- Deep.

The superficial system drains the skin and superficial tissues above the Buck's fascia. It consists of the superficial dorsal vein, which drains into the external pudendal branches of the saphenous veins. The intermediate system lies beneath the Buck's fascia and

Figure 2.4.
Venous drainage of the penis.

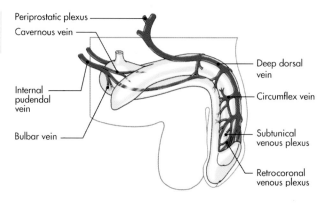

Periprostatic plexus

Cavernous vein

Internal pudendal vein

Bulbar vein

Deep dorsal vein

Circumflex vein

Subtunical venous plexus

Retrocoronal venous plexus

consists of the deep dorsal and circumflex veins. This system drains blood from the glans, corpus spongiosum and the distal two-thirds of the corpora cavernosa. The retrocoronal plexus, made up of veins emerging from the glans penis, drains into the deep dorsal vein, which runs in the groove between the corpora. This blood drains into the periprostatic plexus and then into the internal pudendal vein. The deep drainage system includes the crural and cavernosal veins, which empty into the internal iliac veins via the internal pudendal veins.

Subtunicular veins form a network that drain blood from the erectile tissue within the corpora cavernosa (Fig. 2.5). These venules join to form the emissary veins that penetrate the tunica and drain directly into the deep dorsal vein or via the circumflex veins. The venous network connecting the glans of the corpora spongiosum to the corpora cavernosa allows for the transport of vasodilator substances, that have been absorbed through the urethral mucosa, into the erectile bodies.

■ Subtunicular veins drain blood from the erectile tissue within the corpora cavernosa.

■ A venous network allows the transport of vasodilator substances, absorbed through the urethra, into the erectile bodies.

Neuroanatomy

Innervation of the penis may be divided into autonomic (sympathetic and parasympathetic) and somatic

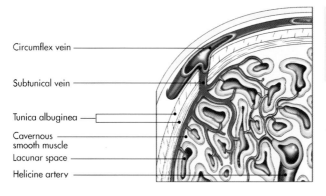

Circumflex vein

Subtunical vein

Tunica albuginea

Cavernous smooth muscle

Lacunar space

Helicine artery

Figure 2.5.
Venous drainage of the penis: opening of the subtunical vein into the lacunar spaces.

(sensory and motor). Three specific groups of peripheral nerves are involved in the erectile mechanism:

- Lumbosacral parasympathetic
- Thoracolumbar sympathetic
- Lumbosacral somatic.

The parasympathetic nervous system provides the major excitatory input to the penis and is responsible for vasodilatation of the penile vasculature and erection. The sympathetic nervous system is responsible for detumescence and maintaining flaccidity. These autonomic fibres combine in the pelvic plexus to form the cavernous nerves, which run down posterolateral to the prostate and into the base of the penis (Fig. 2.6).

Somatic sensory pathways begin at the sensory receptors in the penile skin, glans and urethra. The nerve fibres from these receptors converge to form bundles of the dorsal nerve of the penis; this joins other nerves to become the internal pudendal nerve. Activation of these receptors sends messages of pain, temperature and touch to the thalamus and sensory cortex. The motor pathway to the penis lies within the sacral nerves to the pudendal nerve to innervate the bulbocavernous and ischiocavernous muscles of the

■ The parasympathetic nervous system provides the major excitatory input to the penis and is responsible for vasodilatation of the penile vasculature and erection. The sympathetic nervous system is responsible for detumescence and maintaining flaccidity.

Figure 2.6.
The penile nerve supply.

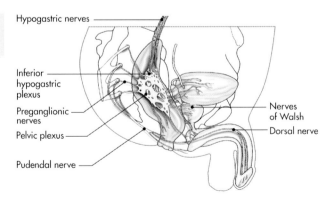

Hypogastric nerves

Inferior hypogastric plexus

Preganglionic nerves

Pelvic plexus

Pudendal nerve

Nerves of Walsh

Dorsal nerve

corpora cavernosa. Contraction of the ischiocavernous muscles produces a rigid erection phase through compression of the engorged corpora cavernosa. Rhythmic contraction of the bulbocavernous muscle propels the semen down the urethral lumen, resulting in ejaculation. It should be noted that the actual deposition of the seminal contents from the prostate, the seminal vesicles and the vas deferens into the prostatic urethra is a separate neurophysiological process to ejaculation and is under the control of the sympathetic nervous system.

> ■ Deposition of seminal contents into the prostatic urethra is under the control of the sympathetic nervous system.

■ Physiology of erection

Initiation

Penile erection is elicited by local sensory stimulation of the genital organs (reflexogenic erections) and by central psychogenic stimuli received by, or generated within, the brain (psychogenic erections). Although the pathways for sensory stimulation are well understood (see above), a variety of stimuli are involved in psychogenic penile erections, e.g. visual, gustatory, auditory, psychic and tactile. Thus, several regions of the brain are involved in the modulation of this type of erection. Reflexogenic and psychogenic erectile mechanisms probably act synergistically in the induction of penile erections.

> ■ Penile erection is elicited by local sensory stimulation of the genital organs (reflexogenic erections) and by central psychogenic stimuli received by, or generated within, the brain (psychogenic erections).

Haemodynamics

Erection follows relaxation of the penile smooth muscle. A number of stages in the process can be described:

- Blood flow to the lacunar spaces is increased following vasodilatation of the cavernosal and helicine arteries.

- Relaxation of the trabecular smooth muscle dilates the lacunar spaces, causing engorgement of the penis.
- Increased intracorporeal pressure expands the relaxed trabecular walls against the tunica albuginea.
- Compression of the plexus of subtunical arteries follows, reducing venous outflow in the lacunar spaces and elevating the lacunar space pressure; this increases pressure within the corpora producing a rigid penis.

The reduction of venous outflow by the mechanical compression of the subtunical venules is known as the corporal veno-occlusive mechanism (Fig. 2.7).

Detumescence occurs through the reversal of this process and follows the contraction of penile smooth muscle. The activation of sympathetic constrictor

■ Relaxation of the trabecular smooth muscle during erection allows increased engorgement of the lacunar spaces, while venous outflow is reduced by compression of the subtunical venules (corporal veno-occlusive mechanism).

Figure 2.7.
The veno-occlusive mechanism of penile erection.

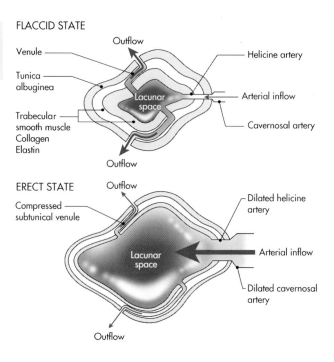

FLACCID STATE

Outflow

Venule

Tunica albuginea

Trabecular smooth muscle
Collagen
Elastin

Lacunar space

Outflow

Helicine artery

Arterial inflow

Cavernosal artery

ERECT STATE

Outflow

Compressed subtunical venule

Lacunar space

Dilated helicine artery

Arterial inflow

Dilated cavernosal artery

Outflow

nerves causes an increase in the smooth muscle tone of the helicine arteries and the trabeculae. Arterial inflow is reduced and the lacunar spaces collapse. Decompression of the subtunical venules follows, as well as an increase in venous outflow from the lacunar spaces. This process returns the penis to the flaccid state.

Neurophysiological control

The overall tone of the cavernosal smooth muscle represents the integrated response to many different pathways and systems (Fig. 2.8). In essence, these can be considered as either:

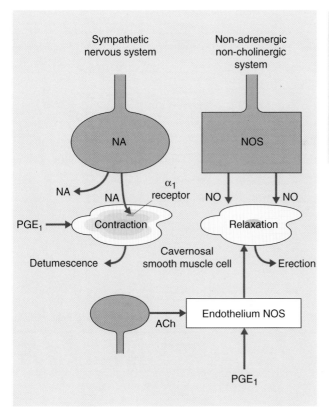

Figure 2.8.
The pathways and systems involved in the regulation of cavernosal smooth muscle tone. NO: nitric oxide; NA: noradrenaline; ACh: acetylcholine; PGE_1: prostaglandin E_1; NOS: NO synthase.

- Extrinsic, involving spinal or supraspinal pathways and classical neurotransmission across neuroeffector junctions.
- Paracrine or autocrine local control systems, involving various neuromodulator substances.

Almost certainly, erectile dysfunction (ED) occurs when an imbalance is created in the integrated response.

Neuronal control mechanisms

As elsewhere within the autonomic nervous system, sympathetic noradrenergic fibres and parasympathetic cholinergic terminals innervate cavernosal tissue. In addition, there is innervation from non-adrenergic-non-cholinergic (NANC) nerves. An understanding of the role of the sympathetic and NANC systems is particularly relevant to the treatment strategies currently available.

Sympathetic noradrenergic nerve terminals innervate both the penile vasculature and cavernosal smooth muscle. Stimulation of this pathway results in the release of the neurotransmitter, noradrenaline (NA) from the nerve terminals (Table 2.1). NA acts postjunctionally on α_1-adrenergic receptors to produce contraction of the smooth muscle; venous outflow increases and detumescence ensues.

■ The neurotransmitter noradrenaline acts on α_1-adrenergic receptors to produce contraction of penile smooth muscle, which results in detumescence.

Table 2.1. Neurotransmitters involved in penile smooth muscle contractility

Relaxation	Contraction
• Acetylcholine	• Noradrenaline
• Nitric oxide	• Endothelin-1
• Vasoactive intestinal polypeptide	• Neuropeptide Y
• Prostaglandin E_1	
• Calcitonin gene-related peptide	

Within the NANC system a neuromodulator, nitric oxide (NO), is released and acts postjunctionally to activate an intracellular enzyme cascade. NO is produced by the precursor L-arginine, which is converted to NO by the enzyme nitric oxide synthase. Within the cavernosal smooth muscle cells, NO increases production of cyclic guanosine monophosphate (cGMP). cGMP decreases intracellular calcium (Ca^{2+}), causing relaxation of smooth muscle; tissue engorgement and erection quickly follow (Fig. 2.9). In turn, cGMP is broken down by phosphodiesterase type 5 (PDE5). Thus, inhibition of this enzyme should elevate, or at least maintain, cGMP levels and restore erectile function.

■ The neuromodulator NO increases production of cGMP, which decreases intracellular calcium, causing relaxation of penile smooth muscle and ultimately an erection.

■ cGMP is broken down by PDE5, inhibitors of which should help restore erectile function.

Local control mechanisms

Various prostaglandins (e.g. PGE_1, PGF_{2a}) are synthesized within the cavernosal tissue. Prostanoid receptors have also been found in this tissue and their activation by PGE_1 has been shown to elevate tissue levels of cyclic adenosine monophosphate (cAMP). Elevated levels of cAMP account for the relaxation of cavernosal smooth muscle and the erectile effects caused by intracavernosal PGE_1.

Another vasorelaxant peptide, vasoactive intestinal polypeptide (VIP), has been demonstrated to alter

■ Local control mechanisms for erection involve the prostaglandins, VIP and endothelin.

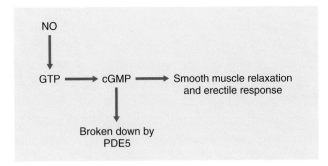

Figure 2.9.
Role of nitric oxide (NO), cyclic guanosine monophosphate (cGMP) and phosphodiesterase type 5 (PDE5) in penile erection.

cavernosal tone *in vitro*. In addition, animal experiments indicate that VIP affects the neuronal innervation of the penis and may well have a neuromodulator role. This would be consistent with the clinical benefits observed with VIP when it is co-administered intracavernosally with phentolamine.

Endothelin, a potent vasoconstrictor, is also synthesized in the corpora cavernosa and has been shown to produce sustained contraction *in vitro*. This, together with their demonstrable atheromatous effects, would be consistent with the role of the endothelins in the development of ED. Certainly, the search for endothelin antagonists (blockers) represents a major current focus of pharmaceutical research.

Cellular mechanism of erection

Gap junctions exist in the membranes of adjacent muscle cells in the penis that are thought to allow exchange of ions such as calcium and second messenger molecules. The major component of gap junctions is the membrane-spanning protein connexin 43. Cell-to-cell communication through these gaps could explain the synchronized erectile responses seen.

■ At the cellular level, smooth muscle relaxation is mediated through two distinct, but interacting pathways, namely adenylate cyclase/cAMP and guanylate cyclase/cGMP pathways.

At the cellular level, smooth muscle relaxation is mediated through two distinct, but interacting pathways, namely adenylate cyclase/cAMP and guanylate cyclase/cGMP pathways (Fig. 2.9). Adenylate cyclase is activated to cleave adenosine triphosphate (ATP) to 3'-5'-cAMP; activation of guanylate cyclase by NO results in the production of 3'-5'-cGMP from guanosine triphosphate (GTP). Elevated levels of intracellular second messengers (cAMP/cGMP) result in the movement of intracellular Ca^{2+} into the endoplasmic reticulum. This, combined with the phosphorylation of cellular membrane proteins which alter the configuration of the voltage-dependent Ca^{2+} channels, causes an efflux of Ca^{2+} from the cells. The overall result is smooth muscle relaxation and penile erection. PGE and VIP, through stimulation of adenylate cyclase, can also bring about the accumulation of cAMP within the cell. Inhibitors of PDE5, the principal PDE in the corpus cavernosum, have been shown to play an important role in maintaining erections through the reduced breakdown of cGMP.

■ Pathophysiology

Normal erectile function is characterized by a delicate balance between vasoconstriction and vasorelaxation of corporal smooth muscle. If a critical level of relaxation is not achieved, there will be incomplete resistance to the outflow of blood from the corpora and a spectrum of penile tumescence will result, ranging from flaccidity to near, but not complete, erection. ED due to incomplete corporal smooth muscle relaxation is termed veno-occlusive dysfunction and may be caused by a variety of aetiologies.

> ■ ED due to incomplete corporal smooth muscle relaxation is termed veno-occlusive dysfunction and may be caused by a variety of aetiologies.

Psychogenic ED

Two mechanisms may be involved in the inhibition of erections in psychogenic ED:

- Psychogenic stimuli to the sacral cord may inhibit reflexogenic erections and consequently the activation of the parasympathetic dilator nerves to the penis.
- Excessive sympathetic outflow in an anxious man may increase penile smooth muscle tone.

The most common causes of psychogenic ED are:

> ■ Inhibition of erection in psychogenic ED may be due to inhibition of reflexogenic erections or excessive sympathetic outflow.

- Performance anxiety
- Depression
- Relationship conflict/loss of attraction
- Sexual inhibition
- Conflicts over sexual preference
- Sexual abuse in childhood
- Fear of pregnancy or sexually transmitted disease.

Vasculogenic ED

The most frequent organic cause of ED is the disturbance in the flow of blood to and from the penis. Atherosclerotic or traumatic arterial occlusive disease of the hypogastric-cavernous arterial bed can decrease perfusion pressure and arterial flow to the lacunar spaces. This results in decreased rigidity of the erection and an increased time period to achieving maximum erection.

■ The most frequent organic cause of ED is the disturbance in the flow of blood to and from the penis.

Excessive outflow through the subtunical venules, despite adequate arterial inflow, may be another cause of ED. In this instance, the perfusion pressures achieved cannot compensate for the unrestricted outflow to ensure adequate penile rigidity. This may be due to insufficient relaxation of trabecular smooth muscle, which may occur in an anxious patient with excessive adrenergic-constrictor tone or in a patient with damaged parasympathetic dilator nerves.

Structural alterations to the fibroelastic components of the trabeculae may cause a loss of compliance and an inability to expand the trabeculae against the tunica albuginea to compress the subtunical venules. This may be a result of:

- Ageing.
- Increased cross-linking of collagen fibres induced by non-enzymatic glycosylation and hypoxia.
- Altered synthesis of collagen associated with hypercholesterolaemia.

The fibroelastic structures can also be altered by surgery or trauma to the penis.

Neurogenic ED

Disorders that affect the parasympathetic sacral spinal cord or the peripheral efferent autonomic fibres to the penis cause partial or complete ED. This is due to the inability of these nerves to cause relaxation of penile smooth muscle. An alteration of the afferent somatic fibres in the pudendal nerve may also lead to ED.

> ■ Disorders that affect the parasympathetic sacral spinal cord or the peripheral efferent autonomic fibres to the penis cause partial or complete ED.

In patients with spinal cord injury, the degree of erectile function maintained depends on the completeness and the level of the spinal lesion. Patients with incomplete lesions or injuries to the upper part of the spinal cord are more likely to retain erectile capabilities than those with complete lesions or injuries to the lower part. In addition, although 75% of patients with spinal cord injuries have erectile capability, only 25% have erections sufficient for penetration.

Other neurological disorders commonly associated with ED include multiple sclerosis and peripheral neuropathy due to diabetes mellitus or alcoholism. Surgical procedures such as radical prostatectomy, cystoprostatectomy and proctocolectomy may result in ED through disruption to the autonomic nerve supply to the corpora.

Endocrinological ED

The growth and development of the male reproductive tract and secondary sexual characteristics are under the influence of androgens, and their effects on libido and sexual behaviour are supported through three lines of evidence:

- Male castrates report a decline in sexual interest and ability, though potency is retained in approximately 50% of men.

- Hypogonadal males have decreased sexual interest which is reversed by androgen administration.
- Antiandrogens, such as cyproterone acetate, spironolactone and flutamide, as well as superactive gonadotrophin-releasing hormone (GnRH) agonists will suppress sexuality in man. The latter may cause complete ED, but sexual awareness and interest may sometimes persist.

Androgens have also been shown to influence the activity of NOS and smooth muscle relaxation in the corpus cavernosum. Endocrine disturbances are an important and potentially treatable cause of sexual dysfunction and include:

- Hypogonadotrophic hypogonadism
- Hypergonadotrophic hypogonadism
- Hyperprolactinaemia.

■ Endocrine disturbances are an important and potentially treatable cause of sexual dysfunction.

Men with hypogonadism have decreased nocturnal erectile activity that often responds to androgen-replacement therapy. Hyperprolactinaemia is associated with low circulating levels of testosterone, which appear to be due to inhibition of GnRH secretion by the elevated prolactin levels. Decreasing libido and ED can be early symptoms of this condition.

ED may also be associated with hyperthyroidism and hypothyroidism. The former is frequently associated with reduced libido and occasionally with ED. The ED reported with hypothyroidism may be due to low testosterone secretion and elevated prolactin levels.

Diabetic ED

Diabetes is the most common endocrine abnormality associated with ED. The main causes of ED are thought to be the vasculogenic and neurological complications associated with this disease. A number of pathological effects of diabetes mellitus on tissue, such as small arterial and arteriole effects, neurological damage (especially to the small unmyelinated so-called C fibres), and sinus smooth muscle deterioration, have all been implicated as the aetiological factors likely to be associated with ED. Diabetic macrovascular complications appear to be related to age, while microvascular complications are affected by the duration of diabetes and degree of glycaemic control.

Impaired autonomic nerve-mediated and endo-thelium-dependent relaxation of penile smooth muscle have been reported in diabetic patients, with maintenance of autonomic nerve-mediated con-traction. In addition, the longer the duration of diabetes, the less pronounced is the neurogenically induced vasorelaxation.

> ■ Diabetes is the most common endocrine abnormality associated with ED and is mainly due to vasculogenic and neurological complications.

Drug-related ED

The mechanism by which drug-induced ED is caused varies with the specific agent and its pharmacological action. Generally, drugs that interfere with central neuro-endocrine control or local neurovascular control of penile smooth muscle are liable to cause ED (see Chapter 1).

Summary

■ The penis consists of three erectile cylindrical bodies: two corpora cavernosa and the corpus spongiosum; the tunica albuginea and the corpus spongiosum albuginea form the walls.

■ The urethra is contained within the corpus spongiosum, which expands at its distal end to form the glans penis.

■ The erectile tissue is comprised of a lattice of vascular sinusoids (lacunar spaces) surrounded by trabeculae of smooth muscle.

■ The blood supply to the penis consists of the pudendal artery that divides to form the cavernosal (main supply to the corpora cavernosa); the dorsal, the bulbar and the urethral arteries.

■ The main venous drainage of the erectile tissue is via the deep dorsal, crural and cavernosal veins.

■ The parasympathetic nervous system provides the major excitatory input to the penis, and is responsible for vasodilatation of the penile vasculature and erection; the sympathetic nervous system is responsible for detumescence and maintaining flaccidity.

■ The erectile mechanism can be divided into a number of phases:
  • Increased blood flow into the lacunar spaces and relaxation of the smooth muscle causing engorgement of the penis,
  • Compression of the tunica albuginea causing a reduction in venous outflow (corporal veno-occlusive mechanism) and an elevation of lacunar space pressure, resulting in a rigid penis.

■ Penile smooth muscle tone is under the integrated control of:
  • Neuronal control mechanisms involving vasoconstrictor sympathetic noradrenergic nerves and vasodilatory non-adrenergic non-cholinergic nerves,
  • Local control mechanisms involving prostaglandin E_1, vasoactive intestinal polypeptide and endothelin.

■ Erectile dysfunction may be due to a variety of aetiologies including:
  • Psychogenic
  • Vasculogenic
  • Neurogenic
  • Endocrinological
  • Diabetic
  • Drug-related.

Chapter 3
Clinical evaluation

■ History

A complete medical and sexual history should be taken during the initial clinical evaluation to help determine whether the cause of erectile dysfunction (ED) is organic or psychogenic or a combination of both. Initial enquiries concerning symptoms should focus on:

- The onset of symptoms: rapidity and circumstances.
- The presence of reduced rigidity or a total absence of erections.
- The duration of symptoms.

Such enquiries are often assisted by the use of questionnaires such as the International Index of Erectile Function Questionnaire (Table 3.1) or the Brief Sexual Function Inventory (see Chapter 1).

Organic causes may be characterized by an insidious and consistent change in rigidity or ability to sustain morning, coital, or masturbation-related erections. It is important to accurately assess libido, as decreased libido and ED are the earliest signs of low serum testosterone or elevated prolactin. Enquiries should also be made as to whether the problem is confined to sexual encounters with one partner or occurs with others as well. The presence of 'situational' as opposed to consistent impairment suggests psychogenic causes as opposed to organic causes. Ejaculation is much less commonly affected than the erection itself, but questions should be asked about whether ejaculation is normal, premature, delayed or dry (as frequently occurs

■ The initial evaluation of a patient with ED includes a detailed medical and sexual history.

■ Organic ED tends to have a slow onset and impairment is more consistent; psychogenic ED is more likely to be situational.

Table 3.1. International Index of Erectile Function Questionnaire

Question	Response options
1. How often were you able to get an erection during sexual activity? 2. When you had erections with sexual stimulation, how often were your erections hard enough for penetration?	0 = No sexual activity 1 = Almost never/never 2 = A few times (much less than half the time) 3 = Sometimes (about half the time) 4 = Most times (much more than half the time) 5 = Almost always/always
3. When you attempted sexual intercourse, how often were you able to penetrate (enter) your partner? 4. During sexual intercourse, how often were you able to maintain your erection after you had penetrated (entered) your partner?	0 = Did not attempt intercourse 1 = Almost never/never 2 = A few times (much less than half the time) 3 = Sometimes (about half the time) 4 = Most times (much more than half the time) 5 = Almost always/always
5. During sexual intercourse, how difficult was it to maintain your erection to completion of intercourse?	0 = Did not attempt intercourse 1 = Extremely difficult 2 = Very difficult 3 = Difficult 4 = Slightly difficult 5 = Not difficult
6. How many times have you attempted sexual intercourse?	0 = No attempts 1 = One to two attempts 2 = Three to four attempts 3 = Five to six attempts 4 = Seven to ten attempts 5 = Eleven plus attempts
7. When you attempted sexual intercourse, how often was it satisfactory to you?	0 = Did not attempt intercourse 1 = Almost never/never 2 = A few times (much less than half the time) 3 = Sometimes (about half the time) 4 = Most times (much more than half the time) 5 = Almost always/always
8. How much have you enjoyed sexual intercourse?	0 = No intercourse 1 = No enjoyment 2 = Not very enjoyable 3 = Fairly enjoyable 4 = Highly enjoyable 5 = Very highly enjoyable
9. When you had sexual stimulation or intercourse, how often did you ejaculate? 10. When you had sexual stimulation or intercourse, how often did you have the feeling of orgasm or climax?	0 = No sexual stimulation/intercourse 1 = Almost never/never 2 = A few times (much less than half the time) 3 = Sometimes (about half the time) 4 = Most times (much more than half the time) 5 = Almost always/always

Table 3.1. continued

Question	Response options
11. How often have you felt sexual desire?	1 = Almost never/never 2 = A few times (much less than half the time) 3 = Sometimes (about half the time) 4 = Most times (much more than half the time) 5 = Almost always/always
12. How would you rate your level of sexual desire?	1 = Very low/none at all 2 = Low 3 = Moderate 4 = High 5 = Very high
13. How satisfied have you been with your overall sex life? 14. How satisfied have you been with your sexual relationship with your partner?	1 = Very dissatisfied 2 = Moderately dissatisfied 3 = About equally satisfied and dissatisfied 4 = Moderately satisfied 5 = Very satisfied
15. How do you rate your confidence that you can get and keep an erection?	1 = Very low 2 = Low 3 = Moderate 4 = High 5 = Very high

All questions are preceded by the phrase 'over the past 4 weeks'.

following transurethral resection of the prostate). The patient should also be questioned about pain on intercourse and the presence of erectile deformity.

Relevant co-morbid risk factors should be identified, such as diabetes mellitus, coronary artery disease, hypercholesterolaemia, hypertension, peripheral vascular disease, smoking, alcoholism and endocrine or neurological disorders. The patient's sexual history should be explored, as this might provide evidence of a congenital problem perhaps due to a veno-occlusive disorder or congenital chordee. Previous surgery, particularly pelvic surgery for bowel, bladder or prostatic malignancy or reconstructive vascular surgery may obviously be relevant. A complete drug history is important since these constitute a major source of reversible ED.

■ Physical examination

■ A thorough physical examination is an important part of the basic assessment.

A thorough physical examination is an important part of the basic assessment for men with ED (Fig. 3.1). Clinical signs of the following disorders should be looked for:

- Under- or overactivity of the thyroid
- Liver failure
- Anaemia
- Hypertension
- Serious cardiovascular pathology
- End-stage renal disease.

Figure 3.1.
Clinical evaluation: physical examination.

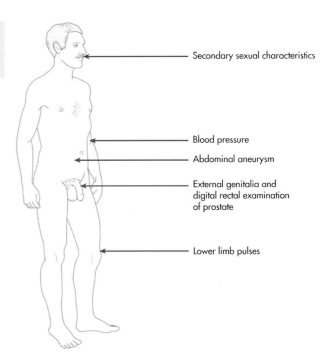

Secondary sexual characteristics

Blood pressure

Abdominal aneurysm

External genitalia and digital rectal examination of prostate

Lower limb pulses

An assessment should be made of the endocrine and vascular systems, the external genitalia and the prostate gland. All peripheral pulses should be measured, as well as blood pressure and cardiac status. The examination of the external genitalia is important as this can assist in excluding congenital or acquired abnormalities of the penis itself. The penis should be carefully palpated along the corpora to check for fibrotic Peyronie's plaques. A number of genital abnormalities are associated with ED including microphallus, epispadias and squamous cell carcinoma of the penis. Small testes and reduced or absent secondary sexual characteristics are suggestive of hypogonadism.

If clinically indicated, prostate size and consistency are assessed by digital rectal examination. Tenderness to palpation may indicate prostatitis. The presence of prostatic nodules raises the possibility of early prostatic cancer.

An overview of the key aspects of patient evaluation is shown in Table 3.2.

Table 3.2. Patient evaluation

Medical history	Sexual history	Physical examination
Chronic conditions	Erectile dysfunction	General appearance
■ Diabetes	■ Onset	and secondary sexual
■ Anaemia	■ Duration	characteristics
■ Renal failure	■ Progression	
	■ Sexual activity (a.m.,	Cardiovascular system
Concurrent drugs	p.m., masturbatory)	■ Peripheral pulses
■ Antihypertensives		■ Occlusive and
■ Antidepressants	Penile sensation	aneurysmal disease
■ Alcohol	■ Pain	
■ Nicotine	■ Numbing	

Table 3.2. continued

Medical history	Sexual history	Physical examination
Vascular risk factors ■ Diabetes ■ Hypercholesterolaemia ■ Familial background	Penile curvature and shortening Altered libido, ejaculation or orgasm	Neurological ■ Penile sensation ■ Bulbocavernous reflex
Pelvic/perineal/penile trauma ■ Penile fracture ■ Bicycling injury	Partner's sexual function Anxiety/loss of confidence	Urogenital system ■ Penis ■ Testicles
Previous surgery ■ Radical prostatectomy ■ Laminectomy ■ CABG	Loss of attraction Relationship difficulties	■ Rectum ■ Prostate
Neurological illness ■ Spinal cord injury ■ MS		
Endocrine disease ■ Hypogonadism ■ Hyperprolactinaemia ■ Thyroid disorders		
Psychiatric illness ■ Depression ■ Anxiety		
Sexually transmitted disease		

CABG = coronary artery bypass graft; MS = multiple sclerosis.

■ Psychological assessment

The determination that the patient's neural, vascular and endocrine functions are capable of generating an adequate erection leads the clinician to suspect psychogenic causes for the dysfunction. The main diagnostic feature for this form of dysfunction is selective ED. The man may be able to produce rigid, long-lasting erections during the night or early mornings, with certain partners, in response to magazines or videos, but not when attempting intercourse with his wife. Underlying relationship problems are a common cause of ED and this possibility should be explored in men of all ages.

Acquired ED

Acquired ED is a form of psychogenic ED that occurs after a long period of successful intercourse. It is more common than the alternative type — lifelong ED. Social changes should be enquired about as a variety of these may precipitate acquired ED, including:

- Health worries
- Death of a spouse
- Divorce
- Relationship difficulties
- Economic concerns.

■ Acquired psychogenic ED may be associated with social changes in the patient's life.

Lifelong ED

Typically, lifelong ED occurs in younger men who have not established their sexual potency. General personality, psychiatric problems and sexual identity should be examined in order to identify the cause of the dysfunction.

■ Lifelong ED occurs in younger men who have not established their sexual potency.

Performance anxiety

Performance anxiety is common to both organic and psychogenic ED and often stems from the anticipation of erectile failure or the loss of erection during intercourse. This phenomenon is disruptive, in that

■ Performance anxiety is often due to anticipation of erectile failure or loss of erection during intercourse.

arousal is replaced by anxiety and inattention to sensation.

■ Tests

Routine laboratory tests can be helpful in confirming a disease process suspected by history and physical examination.

Routine laboratory tests can be helpful in confirming a disease process suspected by history and physical examination. Screening for diabetes mellitus and other systemic disorders, such as liver and renal disease, is important. It is known that the duration and severity of diabetes is related to ED, therefore glycosylated haemoglobin measures (average glucose for prior 2–3 months) may be more useful than a single glucose level. Testosterone and cholesterol levels should also be measured, as well as prolactin, if testosterone is low.

Specialized investigations are performed when a detailed knowledge of the cause of the ED is required. It should be noted that no single test can distinguish psychogenic from organic ED.

Nocturnal penile tumescence

Nocturnal penile tumescence (NPT) monitoring is occasionally valuable for the assessment and appropriate management of ED.

Nocturnal penile tumescence (NPT) monitoring is occasionally valuable for the assessment and appropriate management of ED. As an objective, non-invasive measure of erectile activity, NPT may be helpful in differentiating between psychogenic and organic ED.

In the normal male, three to five erections occur nightly and account for up to 40% of sleep time. The use of NPT is based on the assumption that during sleep emotional factors, such as fear and anxiety, are neutralized, and subjects suffering from psychogenic ED therefore have normal NPT. For patients with organic ED, however, the underlying cause (vascular, hormonal or neurological) does not change with sleep, and abnormal erections persist.

NPT testing

Formal NPT testing may be carried out over two to three consecutive nights in a sleep laboratory. Degree, frequency and duration of penile tumescence are measured using strain gauges. Normal sleep is necessary as sleep erections occur principally during rapid eye movement (REM) sleep. To monitor the sleep pattern, electroencephalographic, electro-oculographic and submental electromyographic measurements are made during the test. Sleep apnoea, which may be associated with ED, may also be identified by sleep monitoring.

The drawbacks of this technique are the anxiety caused by the unnatural setting and procedure, the high costs of the sleep laboratory and the time required. Generally, formal NPT testing has been replaced by simpler methods, such as the Snap-Gauge band technique and home RigiScan use.

■ Formal NPT testing has been replaced by simpler methods, such as the Snap-Gauge band technique and home RigiScan use.

Snap-Gauge band

The Snap-Gauge band is a Velcro band fitted around the penis and worn for three nights. Three coloured plastic film elements are arranged in parallel and each film ruptures at a radial force corresponding to 10, 15 and 20 oz, respectively (Fig. 3.2). The shortcomings of this method are lack of information concerning partial rigidity, number of erections and duration of erectile episodes.

■ The Snap-Gauge band does not provide information on partial rigidity, number or duration of erections.

RigiScan

The RigiScan is a home monitoring device capable of continuously monitoring penile circumference and rigidity (Fig. 3.3). The device consists of a logging unit strapped to the patient's thigh and two loops placed

Figure 3.2.
The Snap-Gauge band.

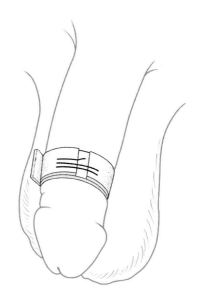

Figure 3.3.
The RigiScan device.

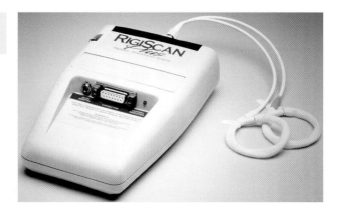

around the base and tip of the penis just behind the corona (Fig. 3.4). To measure tumescence, the loops tighten around the penis every 30 seconds with a force of 1.7 Newtons and the penile circumference (loop length) is recorded. The circumference is measured again after 15 seconds without tightening. An increase of 10 mm or

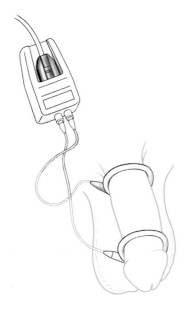

Figure 3.4.
Monitoring of erectile dysfunction with the RigiScan device.

more from baseline causes rigidity measurements to commence. This involves tightening the loops every 30 seconds with a force of 2.8 Newtons. Rigidity is expressed as a percentage; 100% is equivalent to the rigidity of a non-compressible rubber shaft. When the change in circumference is less than 10 mm, the device returns to recording measurements every 3 minutes.

The RigiScan can collect data for three 10-hour monitoring sessions, during which the rigidity, tumescence and duration of each event are recorded (Fig. 3.5). As with the Snap-Gauge band, radial rigidity is measured. Although axial rigidity is the most crucial measurement predicting vaginal penetration, a linear relationship between axial and radial rigidity has been observed. In addition, radial rigidity is functionally related to intracavernous pressure, which is the true measure of rigidity. One drawback of the RigiScan device is that REM sleep is not monitored.

■ One drawback of the RigiScan device is that REM sleep is not monitored.

39

Figure 3.5.
RigiScan recordings.
(a) Normal recording;
(b) subnormal response.

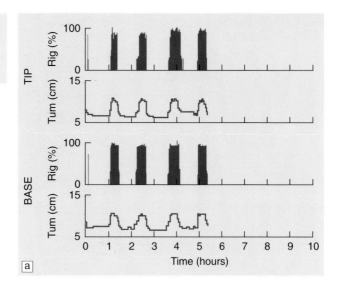

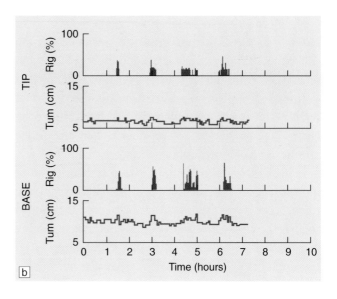

Colour Doppler imaging

Penile blood flow study using intracavernous challenge with a vasoactive agent and assessment by colour duplex Doppler ultrasound (CDDU) is the most reliable and least invasive means of identifying vascular ED. Based on the results of this study, patients requiring more invasive testing can be selected.

■ CDDU is the most reliable and least invasive means of identifying vascular ED.

The choice of vasoactive agent is important. A variety of intracavernosal drugs can induce erection (see Chapter 4), but the two most common agents are prostaglandin E_1 (PGE_1) or papaverine. Phentolamine can be used in conjunction with these agents allowing a reduction in the dose of stimulant required and in the potential penile ache that is sometimes associated with PGE_1 use. If a sustained and rigid erection is achieved within 10 minutes of injection, venous and arterial insufficiency are unlikely. Men with moderate to severe venous insufficiency will have difficulty achieving a pharmacological erection. If a full erection is not seen, or if the erection lasts only a short period, the patient is asked to stimulate himself in an attempt at improving the response. Again, if a good quality sustained erection is achieved, then a severe arterial or venous insufficiency is unlikely. If the response is poor, CDDU with intracavernous injection is performed to evaluate vasculogenic impotence.

CDDU allows the rapid measurement of small blood vessels in low-flow states. High-frequency linear array transducers (5–10 MHz) produce the best images of the penis and emit a pulse of ultrasound that is then returned. When the returning echo has a different frequency to that emitted, a Doppler shift has occurred. The blood flowing in a vessel that is approaching the transducer will produce echoes of a higher frequency than those that were emitted; blood flowing away produces a lower frequency. As blood flow velocities increase, the Doppler shift, displayed as a 2-dimensional colour image, increases. The angle between the Doppler

■ Erections are assessed following stimulation with vasoactive drugs, e.g. PGE_1, papaverine.

beam and blood vessel is important and attention should be made to maintaining the same angle in multiple recordings. For example, arterial velocity in the same vessel will be calculated as 20 cm/sec, 25 cm/sec or 203 cm/sec as the probe-vessel angle changes from 30° to 45° to 85°.

The test itself should be conducted in comfortable, calm and private surroundings in order to alleviate anxiety and thus cavernous smooth muscle tone. The penis can be scanned by a dorsal or ventral approach at the base, with the probe held transversally or in an oblique-longitudinal position (Fig. 3.6). The velocity of blood in the cavernosal artery during systolic and diastolic phases is recorded within 1 minute of injection and repeated frequently until a stepwise evaluation of the entire erectile cycle has been accomplished. A low resistance tissue bed, as in the relaxed cavernosal sinusoids in early erection, will allow forward flow with high diastolic velocity. A

■ The velocity of blood in the cavernosal artery during systolic and diastolic phases is recorded.

Figure 3.6.
Scanning of the penis for colour Doppler imaging.

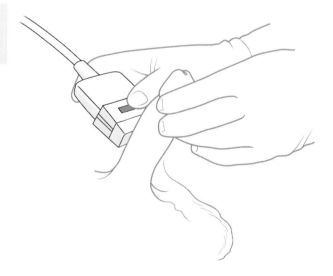

high resistance bed, such as the engorged sinusoids of the erect penis or tonic cavernosal sinusoids in the flaccid penis, will only allow flow during the high pressure systolic portion of the cardiac cycle. During diastole the pressure will be insufficient to overcome the peripheral vascular resistance and the diastolic flow (and velocity) will be low. The patterns produced by a normal patient and a patient with arteriogenic ED are shown in Figure 3.7. The vascular

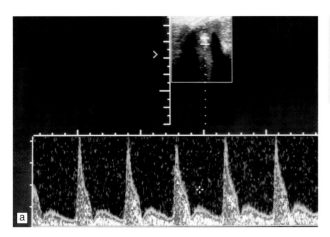

Figure 3.7.
Results of colour Doppler imaging. (a) Normal response; (b) attenuated response.

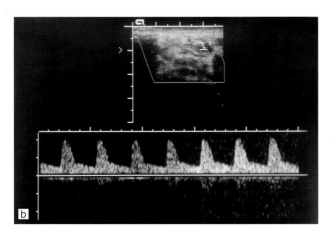

response in a normal patient shows high systolic peaks and negative diastolic pressure troughs. By comparison, the patient with ED presents with low systolic and positive diastolic pressure.

Characteristic patterns can be produced for different vascular-related EDs, such as:

- Failure of initiation (inadequate cavernosal smooth muscle relaxation)
- Failure of inflow augmentation
- Defective veno-occlusion.

With failure of sinusoidal relaxation, there will be no velocity increase. With insufficient cavernosal artery flow, the sinusoids fail to become engorged and the venous occlusive mechanism is not activated. Hence, the wave pattern shows low systolic velocity and elevated diastolic velocity. In comparison, with defective veno-occlusion, both systolic and diastolic velocities will remain high. It should be noted, however, that patients with minimal organic ED do not always show low systolic and high diastolic pressure. Gradations of the two are common and the test cannot be reliably used to discriminate these patient types.

Pharmacavernosometry/cavernosography

Pharmacavernosometry, together with cavernosography, are used to detect the failure of the veno-occlusive mechanism to provide adequate venous outflow resistance. Infusion cavernosometry creates passive veno-occlusion by dilating the cavernosal sinusoids with saline infusion. Vasodilatation with single agents or a mixture of alprostadil, papaverine and phentolamine (Trimix solution) activates the erectile tissues so

The patient with ED presents with low systolic and positive diastolic pressure.

With defective veno-occlusion, both systolic and diastolic velocities will remain high.

Pharmacavernosometry/ cavernosography are used to detect the failure of the veno-occlusive mechanism.

that lower infusion rates are needed to produce an erection. An induction rate is required to initiate the occlusion process, and then a lower rate is used to maintain the erection. The following parameters can be assessed:

- Maintenance flow rate
- Intracorporeal pressure at specific flow rates
- Intracorporeal pressure changes with time after injection of vasodilator
- Rapidity of pressure decline when the infusion ceases
- Cavernosographic localization of the sites of leakage.

An additional issue to be considered with this type of testing is the need for repeat measurements in order to maximize smooth muscle relaxation.

Patients with veno-occlusive defects will require higher induction and maintenance flow rates. In cases of severe defects, erections may not be possible even with infusion rates greater than 200 ml/min (Table 3.3).

Cavernosography using radiographic contrast enables the detection of potential leakage into all penile venous drainage systems (Fig. 3.8). One study showed the leakage at specific sites to be:

- Superficial dorsal vein, 50%
- Deep dorsal vein, 70%
- Cavernosal and crural veins, 70%.

In over two-thirds of patients leakage occurs at multiple sites. The value of this invasive procedure in detecting venous leakage must be questioned in view of the fact that surgical procedures to correct such leakage are not very effective.

■ Cavernosography using radiographic contrast enables the detection of potential leakage into all penile venous drainage systems.

Figure 3.8.
Detection of leakage in the penile vasculature using cavernosography.

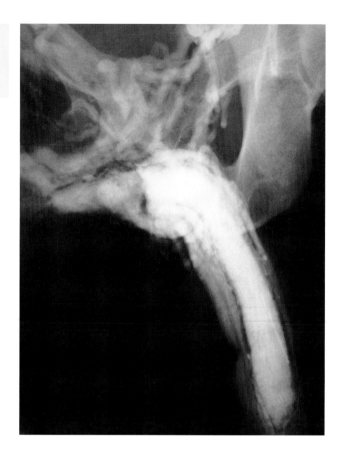

▌ Algorithm

An algorithm for the management of patients with ED is shown in Figure 3.9. The various treatment interventions that can be made are detailed in Chapter 4.

Process	Action	Outcome
Identification and evaluation of ED	• Sexual, medical and psychosocial history • Physical • Lab tests	• ED diagnosis confirmed • Additional testing and/or referral if required
Diagnostic assessment of patient (and partner)	• Review of findings • Patient and partner education • Further diagnostic testing if indicated	• Identification of patient and partner needs and preferences • Referral, if indicated and desired by patient
Modify reversible causes	• Lifestyle modification • Discontinue or substitute medication	• ED resolution with follow-up and reassessment OR ED continues
1st-line intervention	• Oral erectogenic agents • Vacuum constriction device • Psychosexual therapy	• ED resolution with follow-up and reassessment OR ED continues
2nd-line intervention	• Intraurethral erectogenic agents • Intracavernosal erectogenic agents	• ED resolution with follow-up and reassessment OR ED continues
3rd-line intervention	• Penile prosthesis insertion • Other forms of corrective surgery	• ED resolution with follow-up and reassessment

Figure 3.9.
An algorithm for the management of patients with erectile dysfunction. Reproduced from Rosen R, Goldstein I, Padma-Nathan H. *A Process of Care Model: Evaluation and Treatment of Erectile Dysfunction.* New Jersey, USA: University of Medicine and Dentistry of New Jersey, Robert Wood Johnson Medical School New Jersey, 1998.

Summary

■ The initial evaluation of a patient with erectile dysfunction (ED) includes a detailed medical history, a focused physical examination and a psychological assessment.

■ Based on the results of these, a number of investigations can sometimes be conducted, including nocturnal penile tumescence (NPT) testing and the more specialized investigations of colour duplex Doppler ultrasound (CDDU) and pharmacavernosometry/cavernosography.

■ In the normal male, three to five erections occur nightly. NPT is a potential method of distinguishing psychogenic causes of ED from organic causes. This is based on the assumption that during sleep emotional factors will be absent and patients with psychogenic ED will have a normal pattern of nocturnal erections.

■ CDDU is the most reliable and least invasive means of identifying vascular ED and involves the assessment of erections produced following stimulation with vasoactive drugs, such as prostaglandin E_1 (PGE_1) or papaverine.

■ Pharmacavernosometry/cavernosography are used to detect the failure of the veno-occlusive mechanism and specifically, the presence of venous leakage.

Chapter 4
Treatment

Subsequent to clinical evaluation and diagnosis of erectile dysfunction (ED), a variety of management options are available dependent on patients' preferences. An obvious starting point is the modification of potentially reversible causes of the condition. In its simplest form, this can involve lifestyle modification, e.g. stress reduction or dietary changes. In other cases involving an iatrogenic basis for the dysfunction, discontinuation or modification of ongoing therapy can achieve success. More commonly, interventional therapy is needed, ranging from pharmacological agents or minimally invasive treatments, such as vacuum devices, to more invasive procedures, such as penile prosthesis insertion.

■ Lifestyle modification is an important starting point in the management of ED.

■ Psychotherapy

There are three clinical presentations where the physician may consider an assessment and possible treatment for ED from a psychotherapeutic perspective:

- Where significant psychological issues can be identified which underlie the onset and/or maintenance of the dysfunction and predominantly affect the male partner, e.g. depression, work-related stress, trauma. Such issues can all contribute to low self-esteem and a poor self-image.
- Where additional psychological help is required after other treatments have been attempted. An example is a patient for whom Caverject works successfully in

■ Psychotherapeutic assessment and management are indicated for three clinical presentations.

the clinic, but who cannot or chooses not to use the treatment successfully at home, i.e. the patient has the option to regain potency but elects not to.

- Where the patient (or couple) require help in coming to terms with absent or limited sexual functioning, which cannot be helped by further medical therapy. For example, a young man with venous leak or trauma and for whom further surgery is not recommended and other treatment options are resisted.

Additional issues affecting the couple and family group, as opposed to the individual, should also be taken into account. Severe difficulties in the relationship, such as communication problems, hostile and aggressive behaviour and power imbalances, need to be identified and resolved for treatment of the dysfunction to be effective. Couples need to be made aware of the critical role these conflicts may be having in their sexual problems.

■ Psychotherapy is usually only conducted in the short-term and may be used as an adjunct in organic ED.

Short-term focused psychotherapy for ED can be very effective for dealing with identifiable issues that affect the functioning of the individual, the couple and possibly the wider family unit. Longer term psychotherapy would not usually be considered unless the history suggested that more general work was indicated. Psychotherapy can also be used as an adjunct in patients with organic disease. Conversely, organic treatments can be used in psychogenic patients provided therapy is ongoing or has been maximized.

■ Vacuum devices

Vacuum devices work by exerting a negative pressure on the penis, which results in an increase in corporeal blood flow and erection. A constriction ring placed around the base of the penis prolongs the erection by decreasing corporeal drainage. The erection obtained with a vacuum device is different from that obtained normally as there is no relaxation of the trabecular smooth muscle. Instead, blood is trapped in the intra- and extracorporeal regions of the penis.

■ Vacuum devices work by exerting a negative pressure on the penis which results in an increase in corporeal blood flow and erection.

The complete system consists of a plastic cylinder, vacuum pump, connecting tubing and constriction bands. In use, the pump, penis and constriction bands are lubricated with a water-soluble gel and the bands are fed over a loading cone to the base of the cylinder. The cylinder is then placed over the flaccid penis, pushing firmly against the pubis to obtain an airtight seal; it may be necessary to trim the scrotal hair to effect a seal (Fig. 4.1a). Suction is then applied with the vacuum pump to cause engorgement of the penis (Fig. 4.1b). This is predominantly due to arterial inflow, but recent evidence suggests that venous back flow may also contribute to engorgement. After the erect state is achieved, one or more bands are slipped from the cylinder onto the base of the penis in order to maintain tumescence. The vacuum is then released via a valve and the cylinder removed.

The time taken to achieve an erection varies, but is generally around 2–2.5 minutes. The bands should not be left in place for more than 30 minutes, but the procedure can be repeated for prolonged intercourse. A more engorged penis may result from intermittent pumping, i.e. 1–2 minutes pumping, release, then a further 3–4 minutes pumping.

■ The time taken to achieve an erection varies, but is generally around 2–2.5 minutes.

Types of device
Several vacuum devices are currently available (Table 4.1), each using the same principle but varying in the

Figure 4.1.
Use of the vacuum device.
(a) Placement of the cylinder
over the flaccid penis;
(b) application of a vacuum
causing engorgement of the
penis. A constriction ring
maintains erection.

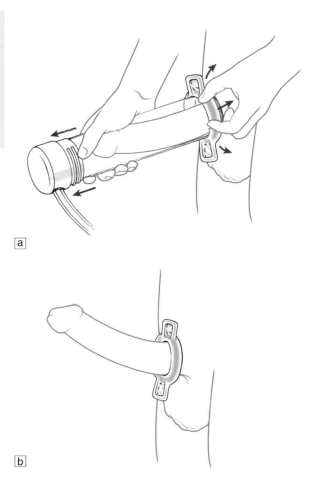

a

b

Table 4.1. Vacuum devices currently marketed

Device	Manufacturer
• ErecAid system	• Osbon Medical Systems Ltd., Augusta, GA, USA
• VED vacuum erection device	• Mission Pharmaceutical, San Antonio, TX, USA
• VET vacuum erection technologies	• Vetco, Birmingham, AL, USA
• VTU system	• Encore, Louisville, KY, USA
• Post-T-Vac vacuum therapy	• Post-T-Vac, Dodge City, KS, USA

method of inducing a vacuum and the type of pressure-release valve and constriction ring. The majority of vacuum devices use either a battery or a hand pump to generate a vacuum. Constriction bands vary with respect to their thickness and grips; shaped bands are available which have a notch that fits over the urethra in order to reduce ejaculatory difficulties and to concentrate pressure on the corpora (Fig. 4.2).

Drawbacks

Patients may complain of pain due to the suction process or the constrictor band. Petechiae of the penis may occur as well as bruising at the position of the constriction band. The band around the base of the penis may obstruct ejaculation, although the development of the shaped band has diminished this problem in certain patients. As the penis only becomes rigid distal to the constricting band, there is a lack of

■ Drawbacks to the vacuum device include pain, petechiae, obstruction of ejaculation, penile pivoting and coolness.

Figure 4.2.
A shaped constriction band.

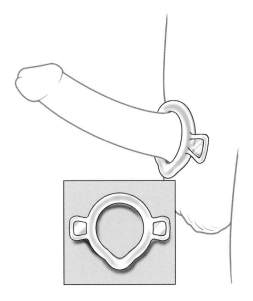

fixation compared with a normal erection, i.e. the penis may pivot at its base. This is known as a fulcrum effect and requires the patient and his partner to experiment with the device in order for the process to be effective. With the decreased blood flow into the penis, the penis may become slightly cool, turn a slightly bluish colour due to cyanosis, and be slightly numb.

The most frequent complaint by patients using the vacuum therapy is the lack of spontaneity, and some partners dislike the coldness of the penis and the need to use a lubricating gel.

Patient selection

■ Vacuum therapy can be used by almost all patients with ED.

Vacuum therapy can be used by almost all patients with ED. It can be considered as a treatment option following the evaluation of the patient's history and physical examination without the need of further testing to determine aetiology. It can also be used by patients failing other therapies, e.g. penile prosthesis, and can produce positive results. Vacuum devices are generally recommended for patients with a veno-occlusive disorder and a 69% success rate is associated with the use of such devices in this category of patient. However, this high success rate is often not maintained in the long-term.

■ The vacuum device is not recommended for certain patient groups, e.g. severe Peyronie's curvature.

Due to complications, the vacuum device may not be successful in patients with the following conditions:
- Severe Peyronie's curvature: restricted movement within the cylinder.
- Severe penile scarring of the corpora cavernosa: penile engorgement may not be satisfactory.
- Severe phimosis: may require prior circumcision.

In addition, the use of the vacuum device is not recommended in patients with bleeding disorders or who are prone to priapism.

■ Pharmacotherapy

Historical perspective

Since the pioneering self-injection work of Brindley, the use of pharmacological agents to produce cavernosal smooth muscle relaxation (Fig. 4.3), and thereby erection, has been used increasingly in the management of ED. Traditionally, vasorelaxant substances, such as papaverine and phenoxybenzamine were administered by the intracavernosal route. However, the use of these agents as monotherapy has been largely discontinued. In the case of papaverine,

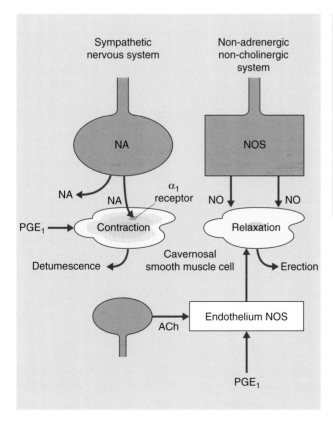

Figure 4.3.
The use of pharmacological agents to produce cavernosal smooth muscle relaxation. Smooth muscle tone is the prime determinant of the degree of erection.
NO: nitric oxide;
NA: noradrenaline;
ACh: acetylcholine;
PGE_1: prostaglandin E_1;
NOS: NO synthase.

long-term administration is associated with a relatively high incidence of tissue fibrosis and/or intrapenile fibrotic nodules. This was most likely due to the acidic nature of the injected solution and has been circumvented to some extent with the use of lower doses of papaverine in solutions at neutral pH, often in combination with phentolamine. Phentolamine is able to block the detumescence pathway of smooth muscle contraction and therefore preserves the erectogenic action of papaverine. In several countries, a Trimix strategy is widely used. This consists of a combination of papaverine, phentolamine and prostaglandin E_1 (PGE_1). In Europe, another combination involving vasoactive intestinal polypeptide (VIP) and phentolamine has been approved for use. At this stage, the worldwide use of PGE_1 delivery systems exceeds all other monotherapies or drug combinations. The salient clinical features of some of the above are described below in more detail.

Prostaglandin delivery systems

PGE_1 is poorly absorbed and is broken down rapidly on entering the bloodstream. This necessitates the use of local delivery systems, particularly intracavernosal and intraurethral (Table 4.2). Another major issue is the stability of the prostaglandin when made up in solution. Harvard Scientific is developing a freeze-dried formulation which may have advantages, but this is several years from being a clinical reality.

Intracavernosal PGE_1

■ Alprostadil, a naturally occurring PGE_1, can be delivered in an injectable form as Caverject.

Alprostadil is a naturally occurring PGE_1 that has been formulated in an injectable form as Caverject. Caverject is thought to mimic the endogenous physiological mechanisms that relax penile smooth

Table 4.2. Formulations of alprostadil (PGE$_1$) used in the treatment of ED

Trade name	Drug company	Delivery system
Caverject	Pharmacia and Upjohn Inc.	Intracavernosal
Edex/Viridal	Schwarz Pharma	Intracavernosal
Icavex	Asta Medica	Intracavernosal
MUSE	VIVUS Inc.	Intraurethral

muscle and induce erection, both by directly relaxing smooth muscle and also by blocking adrenergically induced tone. Caverject is rapidly metabolized, primarily by a dehydrogenase in the corporal tissue, and any systemically transferred drug is metabolized completely within two passes through the lungs.

■ Caverject is thought to induce erection by relaxing penile smooth muscle and by blocking adrenergically induced tone.

Efficacy   Clinical data is available on more than 10,000 men who self-injected Caverject for periods of up to 46 months. In a study of 550 men with ED of various aetiologies, 70% of patients had full erections which lasted for at least 30 minutes following injection with Caverject (5–20 µg). In a 6-month study involving 115 patients with ED, 91.2% of patients reported that the efficacy of Caverject was either good or very good. The general findings from clinical studies are listed below.

• Caverject exhibits a dose–response effect with regard to erectile rigidity and duration of erectile response.

• 75–79% of patients will achieve an optimal dose sufficient for intercourse.

• In-office titration can be successfully transferred to at-home use; the majority of patients (75%) continue to use the dose determined in the clinic in their home environment.

■ Caverject has reported success rates of 70–79%; patient–partner satisfaction is also high.

• Patient and partner satisfaction is high; 73–78% and 72–86% of injections were reported as resulting in satisfactory intercourse by patients and partners, respectively.

Administration   Patients may be offered a trial injection of Caverject to determine the possible cause of their ED as well as to test whether the drug is of potential benefit. If the drug appears to be effective, then increasing doses may be administered until a satisfactory erection is achieved. Medically trained personnel should also demonstrate the correct technique of administration to the patient, as follows (Fig. 4.4):

■ Dose should be optimized and administration demonstrated by a medically trained professional.

1. Reconstitution of the powder form of the drug.
2. The skin over the penis should be pulled taut and the needle and syringe held at right angles to the penis.

Figure 4.4.
Administration of Caverject. Caverject should be injected into the centre of the corpus cavernosum, avoiding the dorsal neurovascular bundle and ventral urethra.

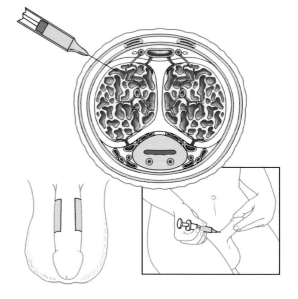

3. The drug should be injected directly into one corpus cavernosum, avoiding any visible veins; the injection site should be alternated between cavernosa.

Dosage The recommended initial titration dose of Caverject for neurogenic or psychogenic patients or in those with unknown aetiology is 2.5 μg with subsequent upward titration in 2.5 μg increments. In ED of arteriogenic origin or due to other organic causes, the recommended initial dosage is 5 μg with upward titration in 2.5 μg increments. Along with this conservative approach to administration, it is recommended that the first dose of drug be given in the office setting. In order for therapy to be successful, as well as safe, patient training is mandatory. Patients should also be provided with written information concerning the steps they should take if a pharmacologically induced erection fails to subside.

■ The initial dose of Caverject is 2.5–5.0 μg, dependent on aetiology, with incremental increases of 2.5 μg.

■ In ED of arteriogenic origin or due to other organic causes, the recommended initial dosage is 5 μg with upward titration in 2.5 μg increments.

Side-effects and contraindications Pain can be experienced and is more likely in patients with anatomic deformities of the penis, such as angulation, phimosis, cavernosal fibrosis, Peyronie's disease or plaques. Caverject may be used in combination with phentolamine to allow a reduction in dose and a decrease in dose-related pain. As with all intracavernosal therapies, corporal fibrosis may occur at the injection site with prolonged use. This results primarily from needle trauma rather than from delivery of the agent *per se*. Priapism may occur, requiring treatment with corpus cavernosum aspiration, intracavernosal injection of sympathomimetic amines, or surgery. Patients should be asked to report any erection lasting for prolonged periods, e.g. over 4 hours.

■ The main side-effects are pain and fibrosis; priapism may also occur.

Caverject is contraindicated in:

- Patients with a known hypersensitivity to the drug.
- Patients with conditions that predispose them to priapism, e.g. sickle cell anaemia, multiple myeloma or leukaemia.

An injectable formulation based on the co-administration of PGE_1 and the α_1-blocker, prazosin, is currently in the early stages of clinical development. Preliminary studies indicate that PGE_1 efficacy is enhanced and as a lower dose is used, induced pain at the site of injection is reduced.

Intraurethral PGE_1

■ PGE_1 can be delivered intraurethrally as MUSE.

In an attempt to circumvent the problems of patient compliance due to 'needle fear', pain at injection site, product stability and cost, an intraurethral delivery system has been developed. Alprostadil has been prepared as a suspension in polyethylene glycol and formed into a small pellet for administration into the urethra via a novel administration system termed MUSE (Medicated Urethral System for Erection). It appears that the distal urethral mucosa is an excellent route for absorption and transfer of vasoactive substances to the corpora cavernosa; transfer occurs primarily via venous channels that communicate between the corpus spongiosum and the corpora cavernosa. The result is haemodynamic alterations in the corpora cavernosa similar to those produced by direct intracavernosal injection.

Alprostadil (MUSE) is rapidly absorbed across the urethral mucosa; over 80% is absorbed 10 minutes after administration. In addition, the drug is rapidly metabolized into inactive forms, such that 60–90% of systemic alprostadil is inactivated after one pass through the capillary beds.

Efficacy   The largest placebo-controlled clinical trial (EASE study) on alprostadil (MUSE) involved 1511 men with complete ED of primarily organic aetiology. A total of 996 (66%) of patients had an erection sufficient for intercourse during the initial in-house titration phase of the study. These responders were then randomized to receive either the drug at an appropriate dose or the placebo for a 3-month period of home treatment. Of the 461 men receiving the drug at home, 299 (65%) had successful intercourse at least once, compared with 93 (18.6%) of men receiving placebo. However, only 50.4% of administrations resulted in successful intercourse. Many of the patients included in this study were postradical prostatectomy subjects. Other authors in less selected series have reported a lower rate of efficacy with MUSE therapy. Studies are now underway to examine the efficacy of a combination of PGE_1 and the α_1-adrenoceptor antagonist, prazosin, in an attempt to enhance the efficacy of MUSE treatment.

■ Success rates of up to 65% have been reported with MUSE.

Administration   The alprostadil (MUSE) applicator is shown in Figure 4.5. The medicated pellet containing a 100, 250, 500 or 1000 µg dose of alprostadil is administered shortly after urination by inserting the applicator stem, which is 3.5 mm in diameter and 3.2 cm in length, into the urethra and depressing the applicator button (Fig. 4.6). The applicator is removed, ensuring that the pellet has been discharged, and the penis held upright and rolled between the hands for at least 10 seconds in order for the drug to be adequately distributed along the walls of the urethra. No more than two administrations should occur in any 24-hour period. Usual onset of activity is 20 minutes and erections may last for 30 to 60 minutes.

■ 100–1000 µg doses are available; usual onset of activity is 20 minutes, with effects lasting for 30–60 minutes.

Figure 4.5.
The MUSE applicator.

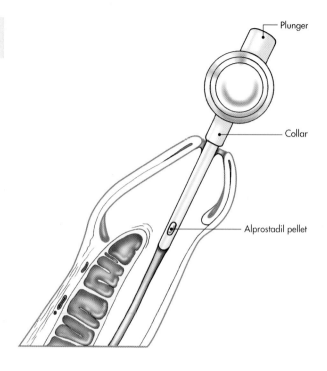

Plunger

Collar

Alprostadil pellet

Figure 4.6.
Administration of alprostadil via the MUSE applicator. The applicator is passed until the collar is at the urethral meatus. The button is depressed to push the alprostadil pellet into the urethra. After removal of the applicator, the urethra is massaged to improve absorption.

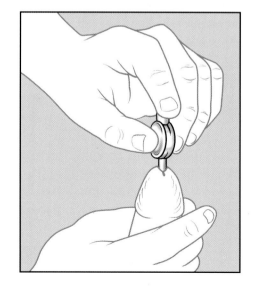

Recently, the manufacturer of MUSE has recommended the use of constrictive rings at the base of the penis in an attempt to increase the efficacy of intraurethral prostaglandin. The rings are applied before the drug is administered and are left in place after erection is achieved. Anecdotally, this is thought to improve drug absorption and transfer from the urethra to the corporal tissue.

Side-effects and contraindications The most common side-effects reported are:
- Aching in the penis, testicles, legs and perineum.
- Warmth or burning sensation in the urethra.
- Redness of the penis due to increased blood flow.
- Minor urethral bleeding or spotting due to improper use.

■ The major side-effect of MUSE is pain; priapism may also occur.

In approximately one-third of patients, the major side-effect was pain and this was the prime reason for the considerable drop-out rate. The mechanism is not clear, but diabetics and patients who have previously undergone radical prostatectomy appear to be most susceptible.

Prolonged erection may also occur and patients should be cautioned about this and about the action they should take. Contraindications are the same as those applying to Caverject. In addition, alprostadil (MUSE) should not be used for sexual intercourse with a pregnant partner unless the couple uses a condom barrier.

Transdermal delivery
Another option to minimize both systemic exposure and tissue traumatization involves administration of vasoactive substances across the skin of the penis. This has an added benefit from the patient's perspective, in being a less invasive therapeutic option.

■ SEPA is a new technology for transdermal delivery of agents such as PGE_1.

Until recently, although various topical agents including minoxidil, papaverine and PGE_1 have been studied, efficacy was found to be limited. However, the pioneering work of Macrochem, using proprietary soft enhanced percutaneous absorption (SEPA) technology, gives ground for optimism. Pilot studies using this gel formulation, first reported in 1996, have been extended. At the American Urological Association meeting in San Diego, Topiglan (PGE_1 in SEPA) was reported to be effective in 80–90% of the 114 patients recruited. Nevertheless, several years of carefully controlled studies will have to be completed, and the issue of partner exposure addressed, prior to approval by the regulatory authorities.

Other intracavernosal drugs
Moxisylyte (Erecnos)

■ Moxisylyte, a selective α_1-adrenoceptor blocker, impedes the action of noradrenaline to produce contraction of smooth muscle.

Moxisylyte is a selective α_1-adrenoceptor blocker that is administered via the intracavernosal route. Its main pharmacological activity is on the sympathetic nervous system. When injected into the corpora cavernosa, moxisylyte impedes the action of noradrenaline (NA), which acts postjunctionally on α_1-adrenergic receptors to produce contraction of the smooth muscle, increased venous outflow and detumescence. As its action on the α_1-receptors is rapidly reversible, moxisylyte is associated with a very low incidence of priapism. Studies show that a high percentage of patients have improved spontaneous erections during treatment and, indeed, that over 50% regained satisfactory sexual activity after discontinuation of treatment.

Vasoactive intestinal polypeptide/phentolamine (Invicorp)

Vasoactive intestinal polypeptide (VIP) has a potent effect on the veno-occlusive mechanism, with little affect on arterial blood flow. Conversely, phentolamine will affect arterial flow without affecting veno-occlusion. On this basis, delivery of both agents should result in an augmented response compared with that achievable with either agent alone.

■ A VIP/phentolamine mix (Invicorp) improves the veno-occlusive mechanism and arterial blood flow.

Invicorp has been shown to be of benefit in an open label study of 500 patients with ED of diverse aetiology. In apparent contrast to intracavernosal PGE_1, a study of 15,000 injections of Invicorp resulted in little or no pain at the site of injection. Intracavernosal administration of this agent has recently been approved by authorities in the UK, Ireland, Denmark and elsewhere.

Other transdermal drugs

Testosterone

Testosterone therapy for ED is indicated only in confirmed cases of endocrinopathies and should be reserved for patients with documented hypogonadism. Currently, the most commonly used form of testosterone therapy is depot formulation of the long-acting esters of testosterone, enanthate and cypionate. These esters are converted to free testosterone in the circulation. Although doses should be individualized, administration generally involves 200–300 mg every 2–3 weeks. Oral preparations are associated with relatively unpredictable serum levels and also a risk of liver toxicity and elevation of serum lipid levels. Transdermal administration has been developed recently. One to two patches containing 2.5–5.0 mg of

■ Testosterone therapy for ED is indicated only in confirmed cases of endocrinopathies.

testosterone applied daily to the abdomen, back (Fig. 4.7), thighs or upper arms have been shown to produce normal plasma testosterone levels. The normal diurnal pattern of serum testosterone concentration can be mimicked by applying patches nightly.

Patients using testosterone skin patches have reported improvements in libido, sexual function, energy and mood. As with other transdermal preparations, adverse skin reactions have been noted in 9% of patients, but these can be treated with topical hydrocortisone or antihistamine cream. Serum prostate-specific antigen (PSA) levels should be measured before testosterone therapy is started. In addition, men older than 50 years must be evaluated for benign prostatic hyperplasia and prostate cancer and monitored during treatment at 6-month intervals.

■ Patients using testosterone skin patches have reported improvements in libido, sexual function, energy and mood.

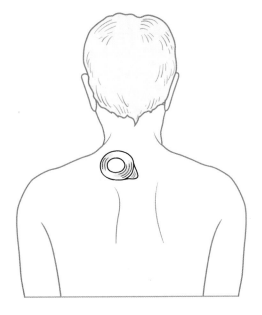

Figure 4.7.
Transdermal application of testosterone.

Oral therapies

The Holy Grail for patient, physician and pharmaceutical industry alike has been the identification of an effective and safe oral agent. A plethora of drugs with differing mechanistic profiles have been used with varying degrees of success.

Sildenafil

Sildenafil (Viagra) is a potent and selective inhibitor of cGMP-dependent PDE5. During sexual stimulation nerves in the penis release nitric oxide (NO) (Fig. 4.8), which in turn causes an increase in cGMP in the corpus cavernosum. Elevated cGMP levels are largely responsible for the smooth muscle relaxation required to produce erections. The drug only works under conditions of sexual stimulation. Overall, therefore, sildenafil acts to restore the natural response to sexual stimulation, facilitating the achievement and maintenance of erections.

■ Sildenafil (Viagra) is a potent and selective inhibitor of cGMP-dependent PDE5.

■ Sildenafil acts to restore the natural response to sexual stimulation.

Sildenafil is rapidly absorbed following oral administration and has a relatively short plasma half-life, both characteristics being important attributes in a drug to be taken orally when required prior to sexual activity.

Efficacy   Over 20 double-blind, placebo-controlled, clinical studies have been completed on sildenafil. In

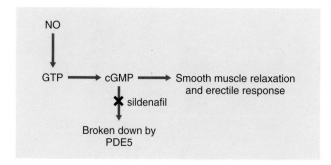

Figure 4.8.
Role of PDE5 and PDE5 inhibitors (sildenafil) in the erectile pathway. NO = nitric oxide; GTP = guanosine triphosphate; cGMP = cyclic guanosine monophosphate; PDE5 = phosphodiesterase type 5.

these studies, the drug has been evaluated in more than 3000 patients, aged 19–87 years, with ED of various aetiologies (organic, psychogenic or mixed organic/ psychogenic). The clinical data show that sildenafil, taken 1 hour before sexual activity, is a simple and effective treatment of ED in a wide variety of patients, including those with diabetes, spinal cord injuries, other co-morbidity and in patients taking a variety of concomitant medication. In most patient populations, 70–90% of patients with ED arising from diverse aetiologies reported treatment-related improvements in erections (Fig. 4.9). In comparison, placebo elicited only a 10–30% response. The sildenafil response was durable; in one 12-month, open-label study, 88% of patients reported improved erections with sildenafil and

■ Sildenafil, taken 1 hour before sexual activity, is a simple and effective treatment of ED in a wide variety of patients.

■ Response rates of 70–90% have been reported with sildenafil.

Figure 4.9.
Improvement in the ability to (a) achieve and (b) maintain an erection, at the end of a 3-month (■) or 6-month (■) study, as assessed by patients using the International Index of Erectile Function (IIEF) Questionnaire (a score of 4 is equivalent to an answer of 'most times' on the questionnaire).

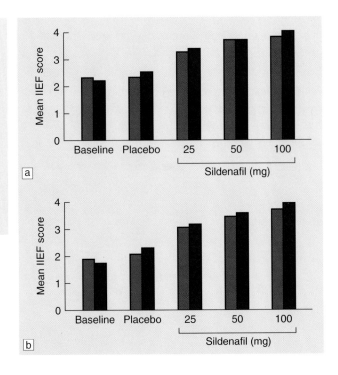

87% completed the study. In addition, 90% of patients wished to continue treatment when available.

Dosage and administration Sildenafil is supplied in tablets containing 25 mg, 50 mg and 100 mg sildenafil citrate. The response is dose-related, with a recommended initial dose of 50 mg, taken approximately 1 hour before sexual activity. Based on efficacy or tolerance, the dose may be increased to 100 mg or reduced to 25 mg. Doses greater than the maximum recommended dose of 100 mg have not been associated with improved therapeutic benefit, but have been associated with an increased rate of adverse event reporting.

■ The recommended initial dose of sildenafil is 50 mg, taken approximately 1 hour before sexual activity.

The major advantages of sildenafil are that erections only occur if the patient is sexually stimulated and that the patient and his partner do not have to interrupt their sexual activity to generate an erection. Overall, this allows sexual activity to return to a natural setting.

Clinical safety Sildenafil is well tolerated with most adverse events being mild and transient in nature. In large, long-term, open-label studies, almost 90% of patients continued treatment, with only 2% withdrawing due to adverse events. In all studies, only 1.2% of patients on sildenafil discontinued it due to treatment-related events, compared with 0.6% of those patients receiving placebo. The most common adverse events associated with sildenafil treatment are headache, flushing, dyspepsia, and nasal congestion/ stuffiness. Sildenafil is also a weak inhibitor of PDE6 and hence transient visual disturbances (subtle changes in colour or brightness perception) have been noted in a small number (2.7%) of patients at the maximum recommended dose. Sildenafil is not associated with

■ Sildenafil is well tolerated with most adverse events being mild and transient in nature.

local adverse events, such as fibrosis or the penile or urethral pain that is linked to intracavernosal or intra-urethral agents. No cases of priapism have been noted.

As well as enhancing the response of endogenous (naturally occurring) NO, sildenafil will also augment the response of exogenously applied nitrates, resulting in profound hypotension. For this reason, the use of sildenafil is absolutely contraindicated in patients using nitroglycerin or other nitrate-based medications. In addition, amyl nitrate, which is sometimes used on a recreational basis, should not be combined with sildenafil.

Sildenafil is cleared predominantly by cytochrome P450 isozymes (CYP3A4) in the liver. Clearance of the drug is reduced in the elderly and in patients with renal or hepatic insufficiency, although dose adjustment is not generally required. Inhibitors of CYP3A4, such as cimetidine, ketoconazole and erythromycin, reduce the clearance of sildenafil. However, any change in pharmacokinetics is not associated with an increased rate of adverse events. Pharmacokinetic studies and analysis of safety data obtained from major clinical trials show no difference in the side-effect profile of sildenafil in patients receiving a wide range of other medications.

Phentolamine (Vasomax)

Phentolamine blocks postjunctional α_1-adrenoceptors, resulting in a reduction in cavernosal smooth muscle contraction and a reduction in detumescence; this manifests as an erection in the patient. However, the effects are modified by its blockade of prejunctional α_2-adrenoceptors causing a rise in NA. Phentolamine also demonstrates some antiserotonin actions and a direct

■ The use of sildenafil is absolutely contraindicated in patients using nitroglycerin or other nitrate-based medications.

■ The side-effect profile of sildenafil does not appear to be affected by a wide range of concomitant medications.

■ Phentolamine blocks postjunctional α_1-adrenoceptors, resulting in a reduction in cavernosal smooth muscle contraction and a reduction in detumescence.

non-specific relaxant effect on blood vessels. Clinical studies have shown that oral administration of a 50 mg dose of phentolamine produced functional erections in 42% of patients with psychogenic and mild arteriogenic ED. Other studies, involving the application of filter paper impregnated with 20–40 mg of phentolamine to the buccal mucosa 15 minutes before intercourse, produced functional erections in 32% of patients compared with 13% of those who received placebo. More recently, two trials have demonstrated an efficacy of oral phentolamine (Vasomax) of 60% when administered 30 minutes prior to sexual activity; however, the placebo response rate was high at 40%, but the approach looks promising.

- Two trials have demonstrated an efficacy of oral phentolamine (Vasomax) of 60% when administered 30 minutes prior to sexual acitivity; however, the placebo response rate was high at 40%.

Yohimbine

Yohimbine, an indole alkaloid, functions as an α_2-adrenoceptor antagonist with central and peripheral effects. Although the drug is used widely in the community and under prescription, little data are available from carefully controlled trials. In addition, side-effects include anxiety, nausea, palpitations, fine tremor and elevations in diastolic blood pressure. More recently, it has been suggested that the combination of this drug with other agents may prove efficacious.

- Yohimbine is an α_2-adrenoceptor antagonist that is widely prescribed for ED.

Delaquamine

Delaquamine, a newer α_2-adrenoceptor antagonist, is 100 times more selective for the α_2-receptor than yohimbine. Unfortunately, although the compound has good oral bioavailability and pharmacokinetics, early clinical data are discouraging, with little or no significant benefit over placebo being observed.

Apomorphine

Apomorphine has direct central dopamine receptor agonist activity and a recently developed sublingual formulation, delivered 20–40 minutes prior to intercourse, appears to be effective in patients with minimal vasculogenic ED. In 12 patients with psychogenic ED, apomorphine administration resulted in durable erections in eight patients (67%). Currently, Phase III trials are being conducted to examine the efficacy of this agent in men with idiopathic ED. Side-effects, as anticipated, include yawning and some degree of nausea. Submission for regulatory approval is likely next year.

Trazodone

Trazodone is an atypical antidepressant used empirically for the treatment of ED; it has both serotonin agonist and α-adrenergic receptor antagonist activity. One study produced an efficacy rate of 60%, although these results have not been duplicated. It is used medically at a dose of 50–200 mg at bedtime. Side-effects reported with trazodone include priapism.

L-arginine

L-arginine is the precursor of NO. A placebo-controlled trial involving the administration of large doses of L-arginine (2800 mg daily) for 2 weeks has been shown to result in improved erections in 40% of patients.

Overall efficacy

Overall, in the absence of carefully controlled clinical trials or other means of objective assessment, none of the above agents, apart from sildenafil and Vasomax, has yet shown reproducible benefit over that obtained with placebo. Safety issues with many of these agents also need to be addressed.

■ Surgery
Venous leakage

Venous leakage, due to veno-occlusive dysfunction, results in decreased venous outflow resistance in the sinusoidal spaces of the corpora cavernosa and consequently in unsustained erections. Diagnosis is based on pharmacavernosometry and caverno-sography (see Chapter 3), which also allow localization of the sites of leakage. Surgery involves penile venous ligation or embolization, which reduces the number of channels for venous outflow and therefore increases venous resistance. Surgery can be considered in any patient with physiological evidence of venous leakage; poor or no response to intracavernosal vasoactive agents; or a requirement for a high induction rate to develop and sustain an erection on pharmacavernosometry. However, patients should be informed about the relatively poor outcome.

■ Surgery for venous leakage involves penile venous ligation or embolization.

Venous ligation restores spontaneous erections in only 50% of patients and is probably a reflection of the poor understanding of the causes of veno-occlusive dysfunction. Long-term improvement is inconsistent.

■ Venous ligation restores spontaneous erections in only 50% of patients.

Surgical procedure

Two approaches can be adopted (Fig. 4.10):

- Ligation of all veins draining from the penis, i.e. deep dorsal vein, cavernosal veins and crural veins.
- Ligation and division of the deep dorsal vein.

Figure 4.10.
Surgery for venous leakage.
The deep dorsal vein is
mobilized and a segment
excised.

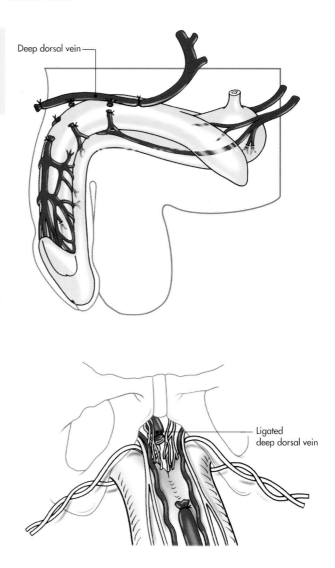

Deep dorsal vein

Ligated
deep dorsal vein

■ Arterial revascularization
is an experimental
procedure used for
treatment of vasculogenic
ED.

Arterial revascularization

There are several treatment options for vasculogenic
ED, and of these penile revascularization is likely to
restore the patient's original erectile function without

the need for additional therapy. It should be noted that this is considered an experimental procedure, suitable for patients less than 50 years of age. Candidates should be neurologically intact and have vasculogenic ED due to trauma not systemic disease. Candidates for penile bypass surgery should be evaluated initially by penile Doppler ultrasound to assess the blood flow in the dorsal arteries, as well as the patency and flow in the deep dorsal vein. The results will determine whether the patient has a functional arterial pathology and should undergo pudendal angiography.

The pelvic angiogram is used to diagnose pathologies in the common iliac arteries or in the origin of the hypogastric arteries, and for visualization of the inferior epigastric arteries (donor vessels) and the dorsal arteries (recipient vessels). Arterial disease may involve any part of the vessel, but the distal pudendal artery or proximal penile branches are more frequently affected. Up to 65% of patients report return of erectile function following arterial revascularization, but careful patient selection is necessary. Generally, good results are only obtained in young men with pure arteriogenic ED due, for example, to previous pelvic fracture. As in venous leakage surgery, long-term outcome is uncertain.

■ Generally, good results are only obtained in young men with pure arteriogenic ED.

Surgical procedure
This involves two stages:
- Mobilizing the inferior epigastric artery.
- Anastomosis between the epigastric artery and the penile dorsal arteries or the deep dorsal vein (Fig. 4.11).

The actual anastomotic site is determined according to the location of the arterial disease identified (Table 4.3).

Figure 4.11.
Arterial revascularization.

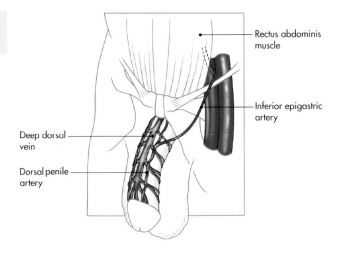

Rectus abdominis
muscle

Inferior epigastric
artery

Deep dorsal
vein

Dorsal penile
artery

Table 4.3. Examples of arterial revascularization undertaken according to site of vascular obstruction

Arteriographic obstruction	Anastomosis	Objective
Distal disease Arterial occlusive disease in the cavernosal and dorsal arteries	Inferior epigastric artery to one of the dorsal arteries	Increase perfusion pressure and inflow to cavernosal arteries retrogradely through the proximal dorsal arteries or through the distal dorsal artery branches to the cavernosal artery
Proximal disease Bilateral focal disease proximal to cavernosal artery in the internal pudendal artery	Inferior epigastric artery to an isolated deep dorsal vein	Increase perfusion pressure and inflow to the corpora retrogradely from the deep dorsal vein through the emissary vein and the subtunical vein
Mixed disease	Inferior epigastric artery to a combined anastomosis of the deep dorsal vein and one of the dorsal arteries	Increase perfusion pressure to corpora from enhanced arterial inflow and increased venous pressure

Complications

Complications associated with these surgical procedures
include:

- Arterial haemorrhage in the first few weeks due to blunt trauma: sexual intercourse is not recommended for 6 weeks postoperatively.
- Glans penis hyperaemia: usually avoided by ligation of the distal end of the deep dorsal vein.
- Anastomotic occlusion.
- Diminished penile sensation or pain from injury to the nearby dorsal nerve.
- Loss of penile length due to fibrosis of the suspensory and fundiform ligaments.

■ There are a number of complications associated with arterial revascularization.

Peyronie's disease

Surgical treatment of Peyronie's disease is only conducted when the disease has stabilized — usually 1 year after its onset. The procedures involved in correcting the defect are:
- the Horton–Devine procedure
- the Nesbit procedure.

The Horton–Devine procedure

The Horton–Devine procedure is used for patients with significant penile curvature or short penises and involves plaque excision and grafting. The initial procedure involves complete excision of the Peyronie's plaque and grafting using dermis tissue. Patients should have adequate erectile function to be considered for this procedure. Recent modifications to the technique have led to increased success. Instead of excision, an H-shaped incision has allowed distension of the area of curvature, over which the graft can be placed. Various grafting materials have been used, including saphenous vein, dura mater, tunica vaginalis, temporalis fascia and Gore-Tex.

■ The Horton–Devine procedure is used for patients with significant penile curvature or short penises and involves plaque excision and grafting.

The Nesbit procedure

The Nesbit procedure involves shortening of the opposite side of the penis using plication or excision of an ellipse of tunica albuginea.

The Nesbit procedure involves shortening of the opposite side of the penis using plication or excision of an ellipse of tunica albuginea. An artificial erection is created prior to surgery using saline or a vasoactive drug and the site of maximum bend is marked with a stay suture. The operation is performed through a circumglandular incision, after which the Buck's fascia is incised longitudinally and dissected to expose the tunica albuginea. The Nesbit ellipse is marked out opposite the side of maximum deformity; 1 mm of ellipse is allowed for every 10° of the bend (Fig. 4.12). The ellipse is excised with minimum disturbance to the underlying muscle of the corpus cavernosus and the correction made is checked by applying two Alliss forceps to the tunica albuginea and reinflating the penis. The defect is then closed with the suture knots on the inside. An artificial erection is induced to check that the penis has been straightened satisfactorily.

Results with this technique are generally satisfactory although one drawback is penile shortening.

Results with this technique are generally satisfactory, although one drawback is penile shortening. Of 359 men studied, 17 had shortening of more than 2 cm;

Figure 4.12.
The Nesbit procedure for correction of Peyronie's disease.

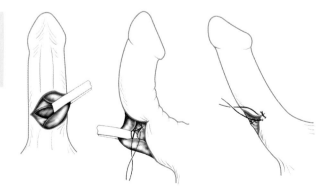

intercourse was possible in 15 of these. Recurrent deformity due to disease progression is unusual and is not generally apparent for 9–15 months.

■ Penile prostheses

Since their introduction some 25 years ago, penile implants are still a widely chosen treatment option, mostly, after failure of all other forms of therapy for ED. Overall satisfaction rate is high, with over 80% of patients and partners expressing satisfaction with the results. Some patients complain of reduced sensitivity and this may be due to changes in the nerve endings following surgery, as tests show that the nerves to the distal skin are generally intact. The erection achieved through the implant will be different to that normally experienced, particularly with regard to the length and girth. Ejaculation, however, should be unaffected. Penile implants, especially the inflatable variety, may need to be repaired or replaced with time and the likelihood of this happening within 5 years of implant is 5–10%. Two basic types of prosthesis are available: semi-rigid rods and inflatable cylinders.

> ■ Penile implants are a widely chosen treatment option for ED, particularly after failure of other therapies.

Semi-rigid rods
The semi-rigid rod prosthesis consists of two rod-like cylinders that are implanted into the corpora cavernosa via one of a variety of incisions: penoscrotal incision; ventral penile incision; dorsal, subcoronal penile incision; or perineal incision. The rods themselves can be either mechanical or malleable. With either of these implants in place, the penis should be worn in the upward position or in the crease of the leg.

> ■ The semi-rigid rod prosthesis consists of two rod-like cylinders that are implanted into the corpora cavernosa.

Mechanical rods

■ Mechanical rods are made up of a series of segments held together by a central spring.

Mechanical rods, such as the Dura II (Fig. 4.13), consist of a series of polyethylene segments which articulate in a ball and socket arrangement and are held together by a central cable attached to a spring. A polytetrafluoroethylene sleeve covers the segments and a thin silicone membrane covers the entire device to prevent adherence to body tissues.

■ The overall length of the mechanical rod can easily be adjusted but the width is fixed, which may be a problem with a broad penis.

The implant comes in two width sizes, 10 mm and 12 mm, and is 13 cm long; the overall length is adjusted by screwing on proximal and distal tips. The size required is measured as the distance from the proximal one-third of the glans penis to the skin over the pubis; this may differ between the corpora but is allowed for in the size of the proximal tips added. Patients with a very broad penis will achieve suboptimal axial rigidity during intercourse with this implant. The Dura II is generally selected for patients with limited manual dexterity, as it is easy to manipulate with no spring-back following bending.

Malleable rods

Four types of malleable rod are available:

- AMS 650
- AMS 600

Figure 4.13.
The Dura II penile prosthesis.

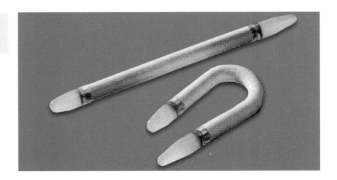

- Mentor Malleable
- Accuform.

The AMS rods consist of a wire core surrounded by a polyester covering and a silicone outer jacket. The 650 comes in two width sizes, 13 mm and 11 mm, and the 600 as 11.5 mm and 9.5 mm; the lengths available range from 12–20 cm; with rear tip extenders providing accurate sizing. The Mentor Malleable and the Accuform consist of a core of silver wire arranged in different configurations. Both versions are covered in a silicone elastomer and come in three widths, 9.5, 11 and 13 mm; cylinder length varies from 14–27 cm and can be trimmed to fit.

■ The malleable rod has a basic wire core, which can be manipulated, surrounded by polyester/silicone coverings.

Inflatable penile prostheses
Unitary inflatable penile devices

Unitary inflatable penile implants consist of a pump at the distal tip, a central chamber and a proximal reservoir cavity (Fig. 4.14); implantation is the same as that used for the semi-rigid rods. Rigidity is achieved by pumping liquid (2–3 ml) into the central chamber from the reservoir. Bending the cylinder will force the liquid back into the reservoir and cause deflation of the implant. The only device of this type available is the Dynaflex. This comes in two widths, 11 and 13 mm and in a variety of lengths.

■ Unitary inflatable penile implants consist of a pump at the distal tip, a central chamber and a proximal reservoir cavity.

■ Rigidity is achieved by pumping liquid (2–3 ml) into the central chamber from the reservoir.

Two-piece inflatable devices

Two-piece inflatable implants consist of two inflatable cylinders inserted in the corpora cavernosa, which are connected to a pump-reservoir located in the scrotum. Two models are available:
- Mark II
- Ambicor.

Rigidity is achieved by squeezing the pump-reservoir to inflate the cylinders. The reservoir volume in the Mark

■ The two-piece inflatable implant consists of two inflatable cylinders and a pump-reservoir.

Figure 4.14.
Unitary inflatable penile prostheses (a). The implanted device (b).

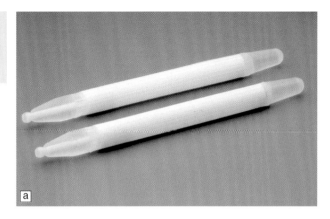

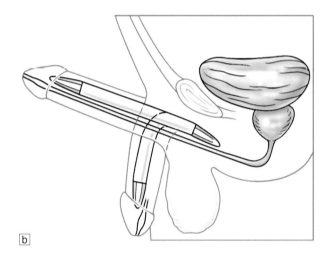

II is 20 ml and this may compromise rigidity or flaccidity in the long or very wide penis as only 15 ml is available for transfer. Due to its size the reservoir is generally positioned between the testicles.

Additional storage is available in the proximal part of the Ambicor device and consequently the pump is smaller and only 3 ml of fluid needs to be transferred between the reservoir and the cylinders. Three width sizes are available: 11, 13 and 15 mm.

Three-piece inflatable devices

The three-piece inflatable implant (Fig. 4.15) is more complex than the other penile prostheses and consists of two inflatable cylinders placed in the corpora cavernosa, a small pump that resides in the scrotum, and a large saline reservoir which is placed inside the body cavity beneath the rectus muscles of the abdomen. A number of three-piece devices are available (Table 4.4). The advantage of this system is that the large reservoir volume allows complete removal of the fluid from the cylinders to generate a flaccid state. In addition, a very large penis can be completely filled. The reservoir may be placed in a suprapubic position or alternatively an epigastric location if the pelvis is excessively scarred.

- ■ The three-piece implant has a large saline reservoir allowing for greater flexibility in size of penis.

Postoperative complications

Postoperative complications with penile implants include:

- Infection: 1–10%
- Mechanical malfunction: <5%.

Perioperative infection is a particular concern in certain patient groups, such as those with spinal cord injury or with urinary tract bacterial colonization and immunocompromised patients (e.g. post-transplantation). Prophylactic antibiotic therapy may be used starting 1 hour preoperatively and continued for 48 hours to avoid perioperative infection. In addition, the wound should be generously irrigated with antibiotic solutions. Periprosthetic infection requires immediate antibiotic therapy and removal of prostheses. Repeat implantation can occur after a period of healing, which is generally 3–6 months.

- ■ Postoperative complications of penile implants include infection and mechanical malfunction.

- ■ Periprosthetic infection requires immediate antibiotic therapy and removal of prostheses.

Figure 4.15.
The three-piece inflatable prosthesis (a). The implanted device (b).

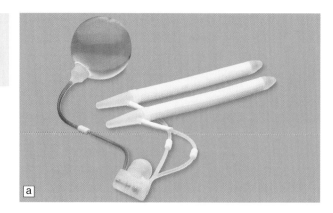

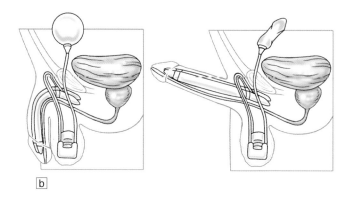

Mechanical malfunction rates have been reduced considerably with improvements in implant design. Eventual fluid leakage, however, continues to be a

Table 4.4. Three-piece inflatable penile implants currently marketed

Device	Features
America Medical Systems • Ultrex • CX • CXM	• Girth and distal expansion: allows for short sizing of penile length and expands with time • Girth expansion only: appropriate in all patients but especially if scar tissue is present or if there is a tendency for penis to curve • Narrower cylinder: more suitable for placement in narrower corporal bodies or those that have penile fibrosis
Mentor Corporation • Alpha 1 • Mentor inflatable	• Bioflex cylinders: more durable and less prone to aneurysm formation; care should be taken with electrocautery due to polyurethane material

problem with many inflatable prostheses and tends to occur most commonly from the cylinders. Replacement of the faulty component is necessary, although the entire device should be replaced if the implant has been in place for more than 4 years.

■ Treatment algorithm

An algorithm for the management of patients with ED is detailed in Figure 4.16.

Figure 4.16.
An algorithm for the management of patients with ED. Reproduced from Rosen R, Goldstein I, Padma-Nathan H. *A Process of Care Model: Evaluation and Treatment of Erectile Dysfunction.* New Jersey, USA: University of Medicine and Dentistry of New Jersey, Robert Wood Johnson Medical School New Jersey, 1998.

Process	Action	Outcome
Identification and evaluation of ED	• Sexual, medical and psychosocial history • Physical • Lab tests	• ED diagnosis confirmed • Additional testing and/or referral if required
Diagnostic assessment of patient (and partner)	• Review of findings • Patient and partner education • Further diagnostic testing if indicated	• Identification of patient and partner needs and preferences • Referral if indicated and desired by patient
Modify reversible causes	• Lifestyle modification • Discontinue or substitute medication	• ED resolution with follow-up and reassessment OR ED continues
1st-line intervention	• Oral erectogenic agents • Vacuum constriction device • Psychosexual therapy	• ED resolution with follow-up and reassessment OR ED continues
2nd-line intervention	• Intraurethral erectogenic agents • Intracavernosal erectogenic agents	• ED resolution with follow-up and reassessment OR ED continues
3rd-line intervention	• Penile prosthesis insertion • Other forms of corrective surgery	• ED resolution with follow-up and reassessment

Summary

■ Psychotherapy for erectile dysfunction (ED) is usually recommended when a specific psychological problem relative to the patient has been identified, in patients who appear unable to use potentially successful forms of therapy, or where counselling is needed to help the patient (or couple) either to come to terms with absent or limited sexual functioning, or with relationship difficulties.

■ Vacuum devices represent one of the minimally invasive treatment options for ED. A range of devices are available that create an erection by drawing blood into the penis. These can be used successfully in most patients with a few exceptions, e.g. severe penile curvature. Drawbacks include lack of spontaneity, penile discomfort and discolouration and coolness of the penis.

■ Pharmacotherapy for ED is developing rapidly and includes a range of drugs that can be delivered by oral, intracavernosal, transurethral and transdermal routes. The most promising agents are prostaglandin E_1 (PGE_1), in the form of alprostadil (Caverject, MUSE or Edex), phentolamine (Vasomax), or a vasoactive intestinal polypeptide (VIP)/phentolamine combination (Invicorp) and the recently marketed phosphodiesterase type 5 (PDE5) inhibitor, Viagra.

■ Surgical procedures can be used, with varying degrees of success, to overcome specific physical problems, e.g. venous leakage, arterial revascularization and Peyronie's disease.

■ A range of penile prostheses have been developed ranging from semi-rigid rods to three-piece inflatable implants. These can provide a high rate of patient satisfaction, although the erection achieved will be different to the patient's normal erection with regard to size and firmness.

Chapter 5
Case studies

■ Case 1: Erectile dysfunction (ED) in a hypertensive man

A man aged 65, married for the second time to a woman aged 47, presents with inability to sustain erections of sufficient rigidity for intercourse. He is hypertensive and is also known to have dyslipidaemia. He has recently been started on a β-blocker and a diuretic by his family practitioner.

Opinion

A careful history is necessary in this case. Does the onset of ED precede or follow the initiation of hypertensive therapy? Have relationship difficulties been excluded? Both diuretics and β-blockers are known to be associated with ED. If these drugs seem to have been a factor in the development of the problem, the authors, after discussion with the family practitioner, would stop this medication. As the patient's hypertension will need to be controlled, an α-blocker such as doxazosin might be appropriate. This compound is associated with a lower incidence of ED than any other class of antihypertensive therapy. Indeed, the incidence is less than that seen with placebo, which suggests a mildly beneficial effect. Doxazosin also reduces low-density lipoprotein cholesterol and triglyceride levels, which might be helpful in this case. As a second manoeuvre, the authors would initiate therapy with Viagra and monitor response.

■ Case 2: Peyronie's disease

A 53-year-old man presents with a 3-week history of painful erections and sudden onset of dorsal penile curvature which precludes sexual intercourse. His past history is unremarkable except for treatment with analgesics for Paget's disease of the bone for the past 30 months. This is now in remission and the patient has no current symptoms. Physical examination demonstrates a normal and healthy middle-aged man, with a normal pulmonary, vascular and neurological profile. Extremity examination reveals a Duypuytren's contracture of his right hand. Genital examination is normal, except for a 2 × 4 cm hard, mildly tender plaque in the dorsum of his penis.

Opinion

The patient is treated expectantly with colchicine and Vitamin E orally for 8 weeks with little improvement. Subsequent injection of verapamil into the Peyronie's plaque produces some softening of the induration of the plaque, but does not relieve the significant dorsal penile curvature. Eighteen months following onset, the patient's pain has resolved, but the dorsal penile curvature continues to preclude adequate coitus. The curvature results in discomfort for his partner and difficulty with insertion. His choices for treatment include expectant therapy or surgical intervention. The patient and urologist elect for surgical excision of the Peyronie's plaque with a saphenous vein graft to close the defect, as his erectile function is adequate and curvature is the principal symptom of his disease. Surgery is carried out and the patient returns with adequate sexual activity, but a somewhat shortened but now straight penis.

■ Case 3: Pelvic fracture

A 23-year-old single man suffered a pelvic fracture and complete dislocation of the prostatomembranous urethra when he fell from a horse 2 years previously. His pelvic fracture was treated conservatively, but the urethral injury required an anastomotic urethroplasty via a perineal approach. As a result of the injury and the surgery required to repair the urethra, the patient now presents with ED. His libido and ability to ejaculate is intact, and he is otherwise fit.

Opinion

The patient most probably has a mixed neurovascular injury which is difficult to repair. The response to an intracavernous vasodilator substance, such as alprostadil (20 µg) (Caverject), should be assessed, as a proportion of such young men will respond reasonably well. Self-injection therapy could then be continued in the longer term. In positive responders, intraurethral prostaglandin in the form of MUSE (medicated urethral system for injection) would be worth trying, as well as the new phosphodiesterase type 5 (PDE5) inhibitor, Viagra.

Unfortunately many patients of this type do not respond to any form of conservative therapy, with the exception of vacuum devices, which are not a satisfactory long-term option in a patient of this age. These young men will sometimes benefit from revascularization using the inferior epigastric artery as the donor vessel. A selective pudendal angiogram should be performed and the option of revascularization or implantation of an inflatable penile prosthesis discussed with the patient.

■ Case 4: Venous leakage

A 43-year-old divorced man presents with gradually failing erections over a 5-year period. The problem has contributed to the failure of his marriage. Blood glucose and serum testosterone, sex hormone-binding globulin and prolactin levels are normal. A prostaglandin-stimulated colour duplex Doppler evaluation reveals normal systolic velocities, but continuous flow during diastole. Dynamic infusion cavernosography confirms extensive venous leakage into the deep dorsal and cavernous veins.

Opinion

This man is suffering from the venous leakage disorder first described by Wespes, the reporting of which was followed by an enthusiasm for venous surgery involving ligation of the deep dorsal vein and sometimes plication of the corpora cavernosa posteriorly. Unfortunately, results of such surgery, even in a young man with normal arterial inflow, are unreliable. Any benefits gained initially tend also to diminish or to be lost altogether over time.

Currently, there is no satisfactory curative treatment for these patients. However, many will be helped by the use of penile rings (with or without a vacuum device), intraurethral or intracavernous alprostadil, sildenafil or a combination of these therapies. Some eventually go on to have implantation of a penile prosthesis.

■ Case 5: Diabetic ED

A 63-year-old married, insulin-dependent, diabetic man presents with complete erectile failure of some years standing. His libido is preserved, as is his ability to ejaculate. He also gives a history of hypertensive cardiac failure, which has responded to treatment with an angiotensin-converting enzyme (ACE) inhibitor.

Opinion

Diabetes mellitus is an important risk factor for ED, as is hypertension. ACE inhibitors can also precipitate this problem, although it is unlikely that treatment with this agent could be stopped because of the risk of precipitating further cardiac failure. ED in diabetes is usually the result of a mixture of neurogenic and vasculogenic insufficiency; however, most cases do respond, at least initially, to conservative therapies. A prostaglandin-stimulated Doppler study would confirm the organic nature of the symptom (even hypertensive diabetic men may develop psychogenic ED) and also evaluate the response to intracavernous pharmaco-therapy. Occasionally, if only a poor response is seen with prostaglandin E_1 (PGE_1) alone, a mixture of papaverine, phentolamine and alprostadil (so-called Trimix) will produce an erection sufficiently rigid to achieve penetration.

If intracavernous pharmacotherapy fails, intra-urethral treatment is hardly likely to be effective. Oral therapy with sildenafil, although worth trying, often does not work in severe diabetic arteriopaths. A vacuum device is probably the best option, although many patients complain of the unnaturalness of the erection this creates and the discomfort on ejaculation. Implantation of an inflatable penile prosthesis is another option, but the patient should be informed that the complication rate, especially infective problems, is higher in diabetics than non-diabetics.

■ Case 6: Psychogenic ED

A 36-year-old man, married with two small children complains of sudden onset ED together with loss of libido. He has no previous history or other medical problems.

Opinion

ED in younger men with no concomitant pathology, such as diabetes mellitus, most often has a psychogenic as opposed to an organic cause. The first question to ask whether the ED that troubles them is situational or constant. Are nocturnal and early morning erections preserved? Relationship difficulties and/or pressures at work often underlie the problem, and are compounded by anxiety that turns presumed ED into a self-fulfilling prophesy. These patients require minimal investigation and maximal counselling support. A trained psychosexual/marital counsellor is usually the best option in such cases, although new medical treatment options, such as sildenafil, may also be of value.

■ Case 7: Neurogenic ED

A 52-year-old married man complains of progressive ED associated with frequency, urgency and occasional urge incontinence. There is a history of syncope and he has a slight Parkinsonian tremor. His supine blood pressure is 130/80 mmHg, but falls to 100/60 mmHg on standing.

Opinion

A history of ED together with lower urinary tract symptoms associated with orthostatic hypotension should make one think of autonomic neuropathy. In the absence of diabetes, as in this case, the most likely cause is multiple system atrophy (MSA), formerly known as the Shy–Drager syndrome. This unusual, but devastating, disease is characterized by selective degeneration of autonomic neurones. Both sympathetic and parasympathetic systems are affected, as well as the pudendal motor neurones innervating the pelvic floor and urethral and anal sphincters. ED may be the presenting symptom and, as in the case with other neurogenic causes of ED, usually responds initially to therapy with intracavernosal/intraurethral alprostadil. Unfortunately, progression of autonomic degeneration is relentless and debilitating; urinary incontinence and postural hypotensions supervene, so that potency problems usually become a secondary issue.

■ Case 8: Premature ejaculation

A 48-year-old single man with a regular partner complains of a life-long history of premature ejaculation. Erectile rigidity is normal and he is otherwise fit.

Opinion

Ejaculation is a sympathetically mediated function, hence the retrograde ejaculation occasionally seen with α-blockers, especially tamsulosin. α-blockers though, are not effective in the treatment of premature ejaculation. A counselling approach can often be effective, sometimes in combination with the use of local anaesthetic gels or sprays to desensitize the glans penis. Recently, it has been discovered that selective serotonin re-uptake antagonists, such as fluoxetine and paroxetine, are potent retarders of ejaculation. These agents may be worth prescribing in certain patients, though they are expensive and carry the risk of side-effects such as gastrointestinal disturbance.

■ Case 9: ED associated with renal failure

A 56-year-old married man with end-stage renal failure, managed by haemodialysis while awaiting renal transplantation, presents with ED. The problem has been gradually progressive, but now intercourse is impossible. Serum testosterone is low at 8 ng/dl and prolactin levels are elevated at 543 ng/dl. Colour duplex Doppler studies reveal a normal arterial inflow and no evidence of venous leak.

Opinion

Chronic renal failure is a well-known risk factor for ED, but the mechanisms for this symptom vary. In this case, the dysfunction could be the result of the hormonal imbalance of low testosterone and elevated prolactin. The normal colour Doppler results rather suggest that this is the case. Before commencing therapy with bromocriptine to treat the hyperprolactinaemia, a repeat serum prolactin should be measured, as anxiety alone can result in elevation of this plasma hormone. A pituitary tumour, such as a chromophobe adenoma, as a cause of genuine hyperprolactinaemia will need to be excluded by means of pituitary computed tomography or magnetic resonance imaging with gadolinium enhancement if the second assay again reveals a high prolactin level. If the pituitary imaging is negative, then a diagnosis of idiopathic hyperprolactinaemia in association with chronic renal failure is likely. The authors would recommend therapy with bromocriptine using incremental doses while warning the patient about gastrointestinal side-effects. Low serum testosterone levels could be corrected by the use of testosterone skin patches, one or two per day. Follow-up is mandatory, because if this therapy is ineffective in restoring potency, the next step would be a trial of sildenafil, or either intraurethral or intracorporeal alprostadil pharmacotherapy.

■ Case 10: Priapism

A 28-year-old black man is seen in the emergency room with a prolonged painful erection which began 12 hours previously. His erection began at night time without sexual stimulation and he reports previous episodes which resolved spontaneously after 3–4 hours. The patient has a known and well-established history of sickle cell disease. Physical examination demonstrates a healthy, well developed, black male with a firm and painful erection of the corpora cavernosa but flaccid glans penis. The remainder of the physical examination is unremarkable.

Opinion

Initially, phenylephrine is injected into the corpus cavernosum followed by the introduction of a 14 gauge needle into the corpus cavernosum and lavage of the corpus cavernosum using a dilute solution of phenylephrine. Dark hypo-oxygenated blood is irrigated free from the penis and corpus cavernosum. The penis becomes flaccid with irrigation; however, within 2 hours the priapism has reaccumulated and does not respond to multiple attempts at irrigation.

The patient is also treated with exchange transfusion and oxygenation for his sickle cell disease without resolution of the priapism.

Despite multiple conservative attempts, the priapism has persisted and the patient is removed to the operating room where a surgical shunt between the corpus cavernosum and corpus spongiosum is carried out through the distal portion of the glans penis. Immediate detumescence occurs following expression of large amounts of hypo-oxygenated blood from the corpora cavernosa. The patient's priapism remains resolved and, although there is significant induration of the corpora cavernosa, healing occurs.

Following complete resolution of his priapism, the patient reports decreased erectile function. Examination of his penis 6 months following this episode of priapism reveals significantly woody induration of his corpora cavernosa bilaterally. Injection of alprostadil into his corpora cavernosa fails to produce a satisfactory erection. Similarly, a nocturnal penile tumescence monitoring study demonstrates no erectile function during 3 nights of adequate rapid eye movement sleep.

The patient is counselled on various methods of restoration of his erectile function and chooses implantation of an inflatable penile prosthesis. The surgical procedure is difficult because of significant fibrosis of the corpus cavernosum. A three-piece inflatable penile prosthesis is successfully placed, however, with excellent function, sensation and return of normal ejaculatory function.

■ Case 11: Prostate cancer

A 62-year-old sexually active man with an elevated prostate-specific antigen (PSA) level (5.1 ng/ml) is evaluated by transrectal ultrasound and needle biopsy of the prostate. The biopsy results show Gleason 3 + 3 = 6 adenocarcinoma of the prostate from two of the six biopsies from the right prostatic lobe. Options for therapy are discussed carefully and the patient chooses to undergo a bilateral nerve-sparing radical prostatectomy.

The prostatectomy proceeds without difficulty and a bilateral, nerve-sparing procedure is performed. The patient recovers uneventfully, with the restoration of satisfactory urinary continence and some erectile function, which he describes as partially rigid, as well as nocturnal erections. His erections continue to improve but the rigidity and duration are inadequate for satisfactory spontaneous sexual activity.

Opinion

The advent of nerve-sparing radical prostatectomy has preserved erectile function in many men undergoing surgical intervention for carcinoma of the prostate. While postoperative sexual function is dependent upon age, preoperative sexual functioning, and the surgical procedure performed, as many as 45% of preoperatively potent men will have some degree of postoperative ED. In this patient, erections were preserved, although they were not sufficient to maintain an active sex life. As a result, additional therapy is necessary to supplement erectile function. Initial treatment with oral agents such as sildenafil or apomorphine is the most conservative method employed. In those patients failing conservative oral therapy, intraurethral alprostadil (MUSE) or injectable alprostadil, moxisylyte, Trimix or other injectable combinations may be beneficial. Patients failing these conservative methods may require a vacuum erection device or ultimately, penile prosthesis implantation to restore sexual activity. Recent studies have demonstrated that early rehabilitation of sexual function in patients following radical prostatectomy may increase the number of patients with normal erectile function in the late postoperative period. This rehabilitation involves injections of intracavernosal pharmacoactive agents two to three times per week to provide erectile function during the healing and reinnervation process. Early use of Viagra is another alternative. While these studies must be confirmed in larger series, it is clearly logical that rehabilitation will increase the number of patients with normal sexual activity following radical surgery for carcinoma of the prostate.

Chapter 6
Frequently asked questions

■ Are impotence and erectile dysfunction the same?

The terms erectile dysfunction, or ED, and impotence used to be considered interchangeable. However, the more appropriate term is erectile dysfunction, which is defined as the consistent inability to achieve and/or maintain an erection sufficient for satisfactory sexual intercourse. Impotence has pejorative connotations and includes this meaning, but also involves reduced potency, which could include loss of libido, being subfertile or not having an orgasm.

■ What causes ED?

The causes of ED are many and varied, and often unknown. ED can arise from psychological problems (psychogenic ED) or can be secondary to disease conditions (organic ED), such as diabetes or atherosclerosis, or a result of surgery. Depression, anxiety, certain drugs, smoking, or alcohol can also cause ED.

■ Is ED like atherosclerosis?

It has been claimed by some that ED could be considered to be atherosclerosis of the penis. Atherosclerosis in the general or systemic vasculature is equivalent to the furring up of arteries and small blood vessels, resulting in reduced blood flow. Doppler flow studies show that this can occur in the penis and in the blood vessels that supply it.

■ What can I do to prevent ED from occurring? (I have normal health for my age, 55 years, but sex is becoming more difficult).

ED is associated with certain risk factors, including being overweight, being diabetic, having abnormal blood platelets, smoking too much or excessive alcohol intake. You can compensate for these by adjusting your lifestyle and so reduce the likelihood of ED occurring. You should also discuss with your primary care physician whether any of the drugs you may be taking could be having an adverse effect on sexual function.

■ Is ED between the legs or in the brain?

Although the end result of ED is certainly seen at the level of the penis, it can arise from changes in many different sites, including the brain and spinal cord. Irrespective of origin, the overall result is generally observed as changes in blood supply within the cavernosal tissue of the penis.

■ I am impotent and drink alcohol heavily, could this be the cause?

This could certainly be contributing to your ED and obviously could easily be resolved by stopping drinking alcohol completely or by markedly reducing your alcohol intake.

■ What is nerve-sparing radical prostatectomy?

Radical prostatectomy is usually performed in the treatment of prostatic carcinoma. There is a danger that during the procedure the nerve supply to the penis may be damaged, either reversibly or irreversibly, leading to ED. To limit the degree of damage, the standard procedure has been modified to maintain as much of the nerve supply as possible. Hence the term, nerve-sparing radical prostatectomy.

■ I am 6 months postradical prostatectomy and get no erectile response to injectables. Will I recover?

It is certainly possible, although not definite, that you may recover. What has been found is that the nerve damage associated with the prostatectomy can improve with time and certainly nerves have been shown to regenerate over a period of 1–2 years. Many patients with ED after this form of surgery respond to therapy.

■ What is Caverject?

Caverject is the trade name for an injectable solution of prostaglandin E_1 (PGE_1) or alprostadil, which is manufactured by Pharmacia-Upjohn. There are other variants of this including Edex, a similar product from Schwarz-Pharma.

■ What are Bimix and Trimix injectables?

Bimix and Trimix are injectables for intracavernosal administration. They refer to any combination, in fact, of either two or three solutions, but usually Bimix would be a solution of papaverine and phentolamine and Trimix would be the same, but would also include a PGE_1 component. Other cocktails are used, mainly in Europe.

■ I am satisfied with my erection after injections, but don't like needles. Should I try MUSE?

Assuming you get a good erection with intracavernosal administration of PGE_1 or Caverject, then MUSE, which is also a PGE_1-containing device but administered via the urethra rather than by intracavernosal injection, may well be worth trying.

■ Does MUSE work?

Although there was much interest and optimism in the response rate to MUSE in 1995, more recent data presented at the American Urological Association (AUA) this year are less encouraging, with response rates only marginally better than with placebo. Pain was also apparent at the delivery site in approximately 30% of patients.

■ What data should I look for to satisfy me that a drug works?

In this era, regulatory authorities including the Food & Drug Administration (FDA) require that in ED and many other disorders/diseases, carefully controlled studies must be undertaken in comparison with placebo. It would be prudent, therefore, to examine the data to see what effect the placebo has. As a minimum, the drug must show superior efficacy, i.e. must work better than placebo. Also, if an existing agent is available, most regulatory authorities now demand that a comparative study using not only placebo, but also this other standard agent, must be used.

■ Prostaglandin injections work fine for me but I get a lot of pain. Is this common and what alternatives do I have?

Unfortunately, it looks like you may be one of up to 30% of the patients who can experience pain at the injection site, particularly at the higher concentrations of prostaglandins. Effective oral therapies have recently become available with the approval of Viagra. However, should you wish to persevere with an injectable, you might try Invicorp vasoactive intestinal polypeptide [VIP] plus phentolamine). It appears to offer a pain-free alternative.

■ What is Invicorp?

Invicorp, like Caverject, is an intracavernosal injectable system. Unlike Caverject, which contains PGE_1, Invicorp contains a mixture of VIP and phentolamine. The data that have been presented look encouraging in so far as Caverject-like erections are achieved, and in addition, there has been absolutely no sign of any pain at the site of injection in over 900 patients; no priapism has been observed. This would appear, at least superficially, to represent an improvement over Caverject. This drug is not yet available in the USA, however, but has been approved by three European authorities.

■ There was a lot of hype about MUSE and then some disappointment. Is Viagra going to be like this?

It is unlikely that the same will happen with Viagra because the FDA have required carefully controlled placebo-controlled studies which have shown that this drug is in fact superior to placebo. The database on Viagra includes over 4000 patients, which is very comprehensive.

■ Is my insurance likely to cover Viagra?

The decision on this is likely to be dependent on your individual insurance company.

■ What is sildenafil? Do Pfizer have two drugs, i.e. is sildenafil different from Viagra?

Pfizer only have one drug for the treatment of ED. Sildenafil is a general descriptor of the chemical that is in Viagra tablets. Viagra is a trade name that can be protected by Pfizer.

■ What is the mechanism of action of Viagra?

Viagra works by inhibiting an enzyme called phosphodiesterase (PDE), in particular, one member of this class of enzymes called PDE5. This enzyme is found within the penis and this accounts for the relatively selective action of Viagra on ED. By inhibiting PDE5, Viagra increases the level of cyclic guanosine monophosphate (cGMP). Elevated cGMP levels result in relaxation of the cavernosal smooth muscle, which in turn results in engorgement of the tissue and erection. In patients with ED, cGMP levels may be low and would therefore be raised by Viagra.

■ Does Viagra affect libido?

There is no evidence to date that Viagra affects libido.

■ Will Viagra affect ejaculation?

Viagra is not known to affect ejaculation *per se*. However, it may reduce the period between detumescence, which is when you go flaccid, and when you are able to have your next erection.

■ What does half-life mean?

A drug that is absorbed into the bloodstream reaches a certain concentration or level in the plasma. Half-life is the time taken for this level to drop by 50%, and it provides information on the likely duration of action of the drug. The half-life of Viagra is 2–4 hours, and the onset of action is approximately 1 hour.

■ Does everyone respond to Viagra?

Unfortunately not. The overall response rate is somewhere in the region of 60–70%, with roughly three-quarters of responders having a full erection. This response rate will depend on the patient population; the response rate in diabetes is marginally less and in postradical prostatectomy, slightly less than 50% of men are likely to respond.

■ I have noticed that injection therapy gives me a harder erection and Viagra a more natural one. Is this a common finding?

Viagra is essentially just restoring normal function and hence you get a natural erection. On the other hand, substances you inject, e.g. Caverject, are having a direct effect on the cavernosal smooth muscle. Also, as they are locally applied, you quite often appear to get a harder erection either subjectively, i.e. as you see it yourself, or objectively when you use a device like RigiScan to measure it.

■ Does Viagra or any other drug cause reversal of ED?

There is no evidence that Viagra does in fact cause reversal of the underlying disease process in ED. However, a number of men are finding that after several doses of Viagra normal activity seems to be restored.

■ Viagra was originally developed for angina. Does this mean my blood pressure will change?

Your blood pressure may change on Viagra, although the changes in blood pressure observed in clinical studies are considered not to be clinically important. If you are on antihypertensive medication you should discuss this with your primary care physician. Viagra should not be used in conjunction with any drugs that contain nitrates, such as glyceryl trinitrate, isosorbide or amyl nitrate.

■ Does Viagra have any side-effects?

No drug is without side-effects. However, Pfizer have worked out the effective dose range that can be used to minimize side-effects. If the drug is used within this dose range, usually 25–100 mg, side-effects are likely to be minimal. Incidentally, not every individual will, in fact, experience side-effects.

■ What side-effects will we see with Viagra?

These are covered in the product information sheet and can include headaches, dysphagia, dyspepsia (a sign of heartburn), back-ache, a little bit of dizziness and some slight visual disturbance (blue haze).

■ My major problem with Viagra is heartburn and pain in my stomach. Is this down to Viagra, and, if so, can I take Tagamet or other antacids to combat it?

It is likely that what you described as heartburn is secondary to a side-effect of Viagra. On consultation with your primary care physician, antacids could be taken, either before or after Viagra, to relieve this pain. It is worth noting that Tagamet will increase the plasma levels of Viagra by 50%, so you may have to reduce the dose of Viagra you take to get an equivalent effect.

■ Does Viagra interact with other drugs I might be on?

Viagra has been studied quite extensively for drug interactions, particularly with regard to diabetic and antihypertensive medications. In general, Viagra does not alter the blood levels of these agents, but must not be taken in conjunction with nitrates.

■ I have been advised that in order to get the best response from Viagra I should take the drug on an empty stomach. What is an empty stomach?

An empty stomach essentially means that you have not eaten food up to 1 hour prior to taking Viagra.

■ I am normal; will Viagra or other drugs for ED enhance my sexual powers?

There is no evidence that Viagra will in fact affect normal sexual function.

■ What does Viagra do for women?

Clinical trials on the effects of Viagra on female sexual dysfunction are underway. In the absence of these clinical results, it would be unwise to speculate as to whether Viagra may have any potential benefit in the female population.

■ If I fail on Viagra what can I try next?

At this point you should consult your primary care practitioner. It is certainly possible that if you fail on Viagra, you may get a response with an injectable, such as Caverject, Trimix or Invicorp.

■ Are there guidelines for ED treatment?

The National Institute of Health and the AUA have been working on guidelines for a treatment algorithm, which has been published as a Process of Care Model.

■ Is there ongoing research in ED or on the reversal of the condition?

This has become an increasing focus for the pharmaceutical industry. Given the drug development timelines and conventional programme, however, it is unlikely that an effective agent will become available for at least 10 years.

■ Will gene therapy be useful in the treatment of ED?

Although gene therapy may prove to be useful in the treatment of ED, it is unlikely that gene therapy will be available in this or any other area for at least two decades.

■ Can I use my injectables intravenously to get better effect?

It would be inadvisable to do this and may be positively dangerous. Certainly with Trimix, side-effects are minimized by the fact that you are applying the drug intracavernously and are, in fact, localizing the effects of the drug to the corporal tissue. To give the drug intravenously would be likely to cause serious systemic side-effects.

■ Can apomorphine be used to treat ED?

A new formulation of apomorphine has been developed by TAP (Takeda Abbott Pharmaceuticals). The preliminary data presented at the AUA this year certainly looked encouraging.

■ Will apomorphine have any side-effects?

Other formulations of apomorphine used in the treatment of Parkinson's disease have been shown to produce quite substantial nausea and vomiting. This new formulation of apomorphine, however, seems to have a better profile, with minimal nausea and vomiting.

Index

oestrogens 7
Spironolactone 7
thiazide diuretics 7
vasodilators 5
history 32
pharmacotherapeutic
  effectiveness data 104
  intraurethral 60–3
  oral 67–73, 100
  self-injected 55–60, 64–5
  transdermal 63–4, 65–6
Dura II penile prosthesis
  (figure) 80
Dyslipidaemia 4

E

Ejaculation 29–31, 53
Emissary vein 15
Emotional disturbances 1–2
Endocrine system
  assessment 33
  disturbances 26, 31
    testosterone therapy 65–6
Endocrinological erectile
  dysfunction 25–6
Endothelin 22
Erecnos see Moxisylyte
Erection
  complete absence 29
  erectile deformity 31
  see also Peyronie's disease
  erectile mechanism 16
    cellular 22–3
    and ischiocavernous muscle
      17
    and parasympathetic
      nervous system 16
  erectile tissue 12
  neurophysiological control
    19–22
    local control mechanisms
      21–2
    neuronal control
      mechanisms 20–1
  pathophysiology
    diabetic 27
    endocrinological 25–6
    neurogenic 25
    psychogenic 23–4
    vasculogenic 24–5
  physiology
    haemodynamics 17–19
    initiation 17
    psychogenic 17
    reflexogenic 17

stages 17–18
veno-occlusive mechanism of
  penile erection (figure) 18

F

Flutamide 26

G

Gap junctions 22
Gene therapy 111
Glans penis 12, 14, 15
Glycosylated haemoglobin
  measures 36
Gonadotrophin-releasing
  hormone 26
Guanosine triphosphate 22
Guanylate cyclase 22

H

Helicine artery 13, 17
Hepatic failure 9, 32, 36
High density lipoprotein-
  cholesterol 6
History 29–32
Horton–Devine procedure 77
Hypercholesterolaemia 31
Hyperprolactinaemia 26
Hypertension 4, 31, 32
  antihypertensive medication
    5, 7
  case study 89
Hyperthyroidism 26, 32
Hypogonadism 26, 33
  hypogonadotrophic
    hypogonadism 26
  hypergonadotrophic
    hypogonadism 26
Hypothyroidism 26, 32

I

Iliac artery 12
Iliac vein 15
Impotence compared with
  erectile dysfunction 101
Innervation
  autonomic 15
  parasympathetic nervous
    system 15, 16–17
  and erectile mechanism
  lumbosacral
    parasympathetic nerves 16
  lumbosacral somatic nerves
    16
  thoracolumbar sympathetic
    16

non-adrenergic–non-
  cholinergic nerves 20
  and noradrenaline 20
  somatic 15–16
International Index of Erectile
  Dysfunction 2, 29
  questionnaire (table) 30–1
Intravenous injection 111
Invicorp 105
  see also Vasoactive intestinal
    polypeptide
Ion exchange 22
Ischiocavernous muscle 16, 17

L

Lacunar spaces 12, 13, 17, 18
L-arginine 21, 72
Libido assessment 29
Lifelong erectile dysfunction 35
Local control mechanisms 21–2
Lumbosacral parasympathetic
  nerves 16
Lumbosacral somatic nerves 16
Luteinizing hormone-releasing
  hormone (LHRH) 7

M

Massachusetts Male Ageing
  Study (MMAS) 2–4, 6
Medicated Urethral System for
  Erection (MUSE) 60–3,
  91, 100, 103
  administration 61, 62
  administration of alprostadil
    via the MUSE applicator
    (figure) 62
  and constrictive rings 63
  contraindications 63
  MUSE applicator (figure) 62
  side effects 63
Minoxidil 64
Moxisylyte 64, 100
Multiple sclerosis 9, 25
Multiple system atrophy 95
Muscle relaxation 22–3
Myocardial infarction 4

N

National Institute of Health 110
Nesbit procedure 78–9
Neurogenic erectile
  dysfunction 9, 25, 31
  case study 94–5
Neuronal control mechanisms
  20–1